Cochlear Implant - Rare and Difficult Cases

Maurizio Falcioni • Giovanni Pepe
Giulia Bertoli • Maurizio Guida

Cochlear Implant - Rare and Difficult Cases

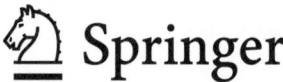

Maurizio Falcioni
Otoneurosurgery and Microsurgery
of the Lateral Skull Base
Azienda Ospedaliero Universitaria
Parma, Italy

Giovanni Pepe
Unit of Otorinolaryngology
and Otoneurosurgery
Azienda Ospedaliero Universitaria
Parma, Italy

Giulia Bertoli
Unit of Otorinolaryngology
and Otoneurosurgery
Azienda Ospedaliero Universitaria
Parma, Italy

Maurizio Guida
Department of Medicine and Surgery,
University of Parma, Unit of Otolaryngology
and Otoneurosurgery
Azienda Ospedaliero Universitaria di Parma
Parma, Italy

ISBN 978-3-032-02322-3   ISBN 978-3-032-02323-0 (eBook)
https://doi.org/10.1007/978-3-032-02323-0

© The Editor(s) (if applicable) and The Author(s), under exclusive license to Springer Nature Switzerland AG 2025

This work is subject to copyright. All rights are solely and exclusively licensed by the Publisher, whether the whole or part of the material is concerned, specifically the rights of translation, reprinting, reuse of illustrations, recitation, broadcasting, reproduction on microfilms or in any other physical way, and transmission or information storage and retrieval, electronic adaptation, computer software, or by similar or dissimilar methodology now known or hereafter developed.
The use of general descriptive names, registered names, trademarks, service marks, etc. in this publication does not imply, even in the absence of a specific statement, that such names are exempt from the relevant protective laws and regulations and therefore free for general use.
The publisher, the authors and the editors are safe to assume that the advice and information in this book are believed to be true and accurate at the date of publication. Neither the publisher nor the authors or the editors give a warranty, expressed or implied, with respect to the material contained herein or for any errors or omissions that may have been made. The publisher remains neutral with regard to jurisdictional claims in published maps and institutional affiliations.

This Springer imprint is published by the registered company Springer Nature Switzerland AG
The registered company address is: Gewerbestrasse 11, 6330 Cham, Switzerland

If disposing of this product, please recycle the paper.

Foreword

Cochlear implantations have become routine procedures in nearly all CI centers. While the surgical techniques employed are largely consistent across facilities, significant challenges arise in cases involving temporal bone or inner ear malformations, as well as sequelae stemming from previous infections, trauma, or chronic conditions such as otosclerosis. Consequently, it is essential for all CI surgeons to understand how to identify these issues on CT and/or MRI during preoperative planning.

This book has been authored by a highly experienced otologist and lateral skull base surgeon with decades of expertise in cochlear implantations. By learning from both the mistakes of others and their own, the author has developed a concept that minimizes unexpected complications. In contrast, being well-prepared and knowing how to navigate challenging situations distinguishes an occasional CI surgeon from a highly skilled otologic surgeon.

Each chapter effectively addresses specific problems, detailing how to recognize and ultimately resolve them. The concept of subtotal petrosectomy, originally described by Prof. U. Fisch in his renowned Skull Base book, remains a crucial approach for many of these scenarios. Although this technique may require an additional two hours in the operating room, the rewarding outcomes and long-term benefits justify the extra effort.

I commend the authors for creating a comprehensive "cookbook" that covers both common and more rare situations encountered in CI centers, often on a monthly basis. As such, this book should be readily available in the operating room or library of every CI center, or at the very least, accessible online for CI surgeons.

Enjoy its content!

Chairman Department of Otorhinolaryngology Thomas Linder
Head- & Neck Surgery
Luzerner Kantonsspital und University of Lucerne
Luzern, Switzerland

Preface

Many possible difficulties may be encountered when facing a cochlear implant (CI): the indications are not always so obvious, some patients are afflicted by medical problems with consequent anesthesiological risks, implant mapping may require different strategies and many different attempts, and even logopedic rehabilitation can be particularly demanding, especially when managing young children or patients with additional neurological comorbidities. However, this book is mainly focused on cases presenting "surgical" difficulties. In such a situation, every single case must be evaluated in depth, especially from a radiological point of view, in order to anticipate the critical points to be encountered during the surgery. Treatment of these cases needs surgical skill; as a consequence, the book is targeted to surgeons with already experience in the fields of standard cochlear implantation and otologic surgery.

After a short introduction on surgical anatomy and preoperative radiological examinations (Chaps. 1 and 2), the surgical steps of the subtotal petrosectomy (SP), with its specific adaptation to the cochlear implant surgery, will be explained in Chap. 3. In fact, SP represents the approach favored by the authors in the majority of the difficult situations, due to multiple advantages consisting in the complete anatomical control, the enhanced light in the operating field, the easier access to the promontorium in case an aggressive drilling is required, and the possibility to completely seal the implant from the external environment. Technically, it is even possible to switch from the standard technique to the SP during the surgery, if the patient has been correctly informed of this option (two cases in the author's experience).

The following chapters will discuss a list of specific situations, namely anatomical variations (Chap. 4), otosclerosis (Chap. 5), labyrinthitis and meningitis (Chap. 6), simple chronic otitis (Chap. 7), cholesteatoma (Chap. 8), previous CWD (Chap. 9), ear malformations (Chap. 10), temporal bone fractures (Chap. 11), vestibular schwannoma and neurofibromatosis 2 (Chap. 12), and rare situations (Chap. 13). Every single chapter will include a brief general introduction, underlining the main problems to be solved in the specific situation, and a list of clinical cases, to better illustrate the different situations to be managed. The majority of the cases will include pictures of the most significant preoperative scans, as well as the main surgical steps, the postoperative scans, and, when considered interesting for the case itself, some postoperative electrophysiological details. The last chapter (Chap. 14) will be reserved for a brief overview of the specific follow-up and the possible complications; the surgical management of these latter will be reserved for another book.

In the majority of the cases, the operating setup necessary for these specific situations does not differ from the standard CI/otologic surgery, which in the author's hands is represented by a last-generation operative microscope, a high-speed drill, an electromyographic monitoring of the facial nerve, and a precise and delicate bipolar coagulation system.

In addition, often these specific situations may require arrays different from the standard ones, to be matched with the special requirements of that cochlea.

Parma, Italy
Maurizio Falcioni
Giovanni Pepe
Giulia Bertoli
Maurizio Guida

Acknowledgments

The authors want to thank Leica for the technical support. All the microscopic pictures have been taken with a Leica M525F20 microscope, a Leica camera HDC-100, and a recorder Hevolution HD

Competing Interests The authors have no competing interests to declare that are relevant to the content of this manuscript.

Contents

1	**Temporal Bone Anatomy Related to Cochlear Implant Surgery**	1
	References	4
2	**Cochlear Implant Surgery: From Standard Approaches to Subtotal Petrosectomy**	5
	2.1 Standard Transmastoid Surgery	5
	2.2 Subtotal Petrosectomy	6
	References	16
3	**Preoperative Temporal Bone Imaging in Cochlear Implant Surgery**	17
	3.1 Magnetic Resonance Imaging	17
	3.2 Computed Tomography	20
	References	25
4	**Variations of the Temporal Bone Anatomy with Surgical Implication for Cochlear Implant Surgery**	27
	References	40
5	**Cochlear Implantation in Advanced Otosclerosis**	41
	References	59
6	**Cochlear Implantation in Post-meningitis and Post-labyrinthitis Deafness**	61
	References	76
7	**Simple Chronic Otitis and Cochlear Implantation**	77
	References	82
8	**Cochlear Implant Surgery in the Context of Cholesteatoma**	83
	References	94
9	**Surgical Considerations for Cochlear Implant Placement After Canal Wall-Down Tympanoplasty**	95
	References	100

10	**Cochlear Implants in Ear Malformations: Surgical Strategy** 101	
	References. 117	
11	**Temporal Bone Fractures and Otic Capsule Involvement: Surgical Tips in Cochlear Implantation** 119	
	References. 130	
12	**Vestibular Schwannomas and Intracoclear Schwannomas: Critical Factors in Cochlear Implantation** 131	
	12.1 Intracochlear Schwannomas 134	
	References. 143	
13	**Cochlear Implant Positioning in Atypical Otological Scenarios**...... 145	
	References. 157	
14	**Long-Term Follow-Up and Complication Management After Cochlear Implantation in Complex Otologic Cases**. 159	
	14.1 Follow-Up 159	
	14.2 Complications 164	
	References. 172	

Abbreviations

ABI	auditory brainstem implant
CSF	cerebrospinal fluid
CWD	canal wall-down
CWU	canal wall-up
CI	cochlear implant
EAC	external auditory canal
EABR	electrical auditory brainstem responses
FN	facial nerve
IAC	internal auditory canal
JB	jugular bulb
LSC	lateral semicircular canal.
MCF	middle cranial fossa
NF2	neurofibromatosis type 2
OW	oval window
RW	round window
SP	subtotal petrosectomy
SS	sigmoid sinus
TM	tympanic membrane

Temporal Bone Anatomy Related to Cochlear Implant Surgery

Deep knowledge of surgical anatomy of temporal bone is fundamental to manage and treat difficult cases of cochlear implant. [1] Often these cases require an approach different from the standard transmastoid posterior tympanotomy (Fig. 1.1), mainly the subtotal petrosectomy (SP) (Fig. 1.2) [2–5]. In this chapter, temporal bone dissection pictures will underline the differences in between the latter and the standard transmastoid approach. Anatomical details of the cochlea (Fig. 1.3) as well the relationship with the carotid artery (Fig. 1.4) will also be described.

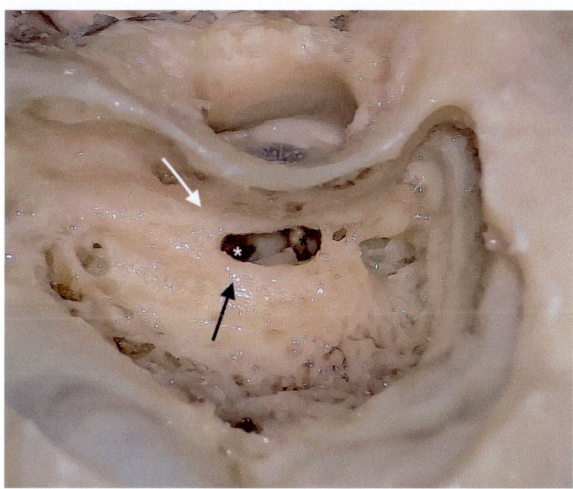

Fig. 1.1 Classic visualization of the round window (white asterisk) area through the standard approach (transmastoid + posterior tympanotomy). The posterior tympanotomy consists of a corridor between the third portion of facial nerve (black arrow), posteriorly, and the posterior wall of the EAC, anteriorly, to access to tympanic cavity from the mastoid. Whenever possible, the chorda tympany nerve (white arrow) must be preserved and represents the lateral extension of the tympanotomy. The stapes (black asterisk) and the promontory are visible superiorly to the round window niche

© The Author(s), under exclusive license to Springer Nature Switzerland AG 2025
M. Falcioni et al., *Cochlear Implant - Rare and Difficult Cases*,
https://doi.org/10.1007/978-3-032-02323-0_1

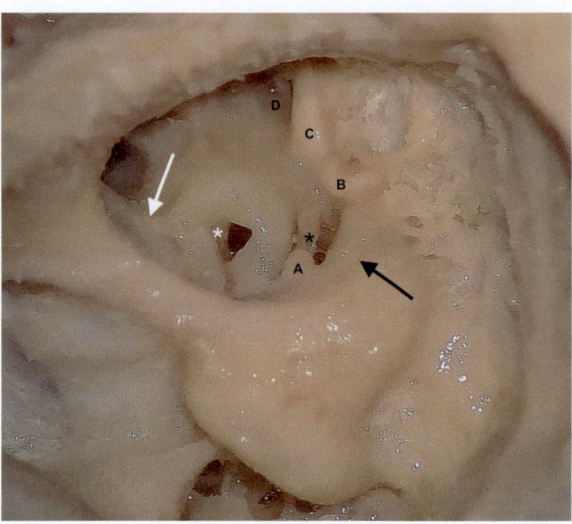

Fig. 1.2 Subtotal petrosectomy. In SP all the external auditory canal, tympanic membrane, malleus and incus are removed, as well as accessible pneumatization of the temporal bone. This allows a complete control of all the mastoid and the middle ear cleft, including an unobstructed view of the round window area, the main target of the cochlear implant surgery. On the promontory the Jacobson's nerve can be identified. The jugular bulb (white arrow), pyramidal process (A), stapedial tendon (black asterisk), facial nerve (tympanic portion) (black arrow), cochleariform process (B), tensor tympany muscle (C) and the tympanic orifice of the Eustachian tube (D) are the other structures clearly in view; each of them may be of extreme importance in situations where it is difficult to remain correctly oriented. The round window (Scarpa) membrane (white asterisk) is partially covered by the overhanging bony borders of the niche, that from the superior margin extend anteriorly and posteriorly. This bony overhang usually partially obscures a direct visualization of the membrane. Sometimes a so-called false membrane, composed by a mucosal layer, occludes the lateral aspect of the RW niche. Correct exposure of the RW membrane requires drilling of the overhanging bony borders, till the complete circumference of the membrane is under control

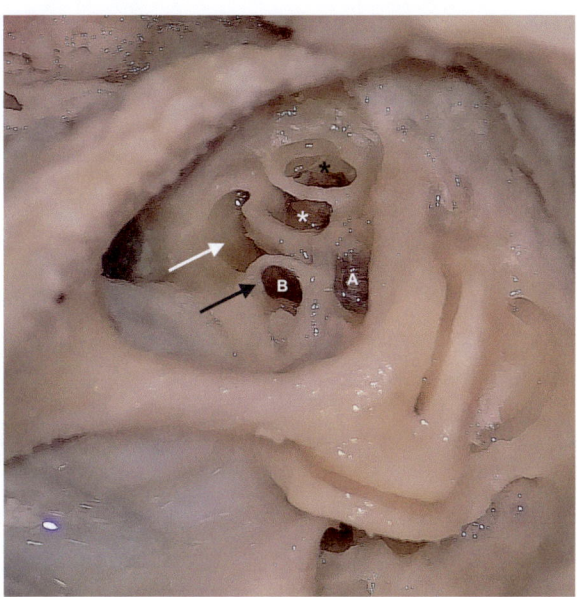

Fig. 1.3 Cochlea. The subtotal petrosectomy allows the possibility to drill the lateral portion of the cochlea maintaining the modiolus that contains the fibers of the auditory nerve. From the modiolus arises a tiny bony structure, called lamina spirale, that together with the basilar membrane and the cochlear duct divides every cochlear turn in the scala tympani (inferiorly) and the scala vestibuli (superiorly). The oval window (A) is directly in communication with the scala vestibuli, while the round window (B) communicates with the scala tympani. It is important to underline the orientation of the basilar membrane to know how to correctly insert the array of the cochlear implant. The initial portion of the scala tympani (white arrow) in fact runs antero-inferiorly to progressively bend antero-superiorly. The inferior border of the round window niche is represented by a bony ridge called crista fenestrae (black arrow). This overhanging bone partially obstructs the direct access to the lumen of the scala tympani. Even if not required when selecting a thin atraumatic array, drilling of the crista may be suggested when inserting a standard/rigid array. The middle turn of the cochlea (white asterisk) lies anterior to the stapes while the apical turn (black asterisk) is located deeply to the cochleariform process and cannot be completely accessed without anterior dislocation/removal of the tensor tympani muscle. It is also important to know that, due to the cochlea inclination, the scala tympani in the middle turn is partially hidden by the presence of the scala vestibuli of the basal turn, lateral to it, and cannot be accessed without a previous drilling of the latter. The close relationship between superior portion of the middle and apical turns and the tympanic segment of the facial nerve is also clearly in view

Fig. 1.4 Carotid artery. The carotid artery (black asterisk) runs very close to the cochlea (white asterisk), a mean 1–2 mm anteriorly to it. The anatomical relationship between the two structures should be well known in order to avoid any carotid damage during an aggressive drill-out of the basal turn

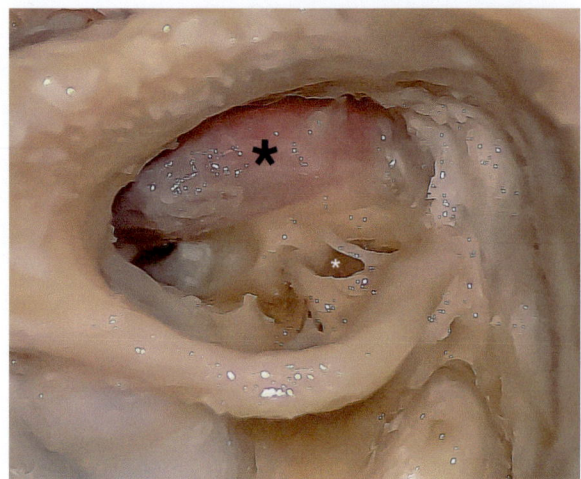

References

1. Sanna M. Surgery for cochlear and other auditory implants, 2015. Stuttgart: Thieme; 2015.
2. D'Angelo G, et al. Subtotal petrosectomy and cochlear implantation. Acta Otorhinolaryngologica Italica. 2020;40(6):450–6. https://doi.org/10.14639/0392-100x-n0931.
3. Issing PR, Schonermark MP, Winkelmann S, Kempf HG, Ernst A. Cochlear implantation in patients with chronic otitis: indications for subtotal petrosectomy and obliteration of the middle ear. Skull Base Surg. 1998;8:127–31.
4. Coker NJ, Jenkins HA, Fisch U. Obliteration of the middle ear and mastoid cleft in subtotal petrosectomy: indications, technique, and results. Ann Otol Rhinol Laryngol. 1986;95:5.
5. Pepe G, Franzini S, Guida M, Falcioni M. Subtotal petrosectomy and cochlear implantation: revision surgery. Am J Otolaryngol. 2022;43(3):103333. https://doi.org/10.1016/j.amjoto.2021.103333.

Cochlear Implant Surgery: From Standard Approaches to Subtotal Petrosectomy

2

The authors take for granted that the readers perfectly know every step of the standard transmastoid approach, so only a few details will be remarked. On the contrary, the subtotal petrosectomy (SP), the alternative approach adopted in the majority of ears with extra-difficulties, will be described in details.

2.1 Standard Transmastoid Surgery

The posterior tympanotomy represents the access to the tympanic cavity and to the promontory (Figs. 2.1 and 2.2). It is important to enlarge it inferiorly, trying not to damage the chorda tympani, to have as much space and light as possible to access the round window. Sometimes the round window is posteriorly positioned and not very easy to be visualized. In this situation, it is very important to correctly skeletonize the facial nerve, even for surgeons that do not identify it routinely, in order to achieve a correct exposure.

Through the posterior tympanotomy, stapes, stapedial tendon, and the round window (RW) should be visible. The RW is a natural access to the tympanic scala. Drilling the RW niche is important to completely expose the Scarpa's membrane. Sometimes the real membrane is covered by false membrane of mucosa. It is more infero-lateral than the real one and is easily removed with little hook to expose the Scarpa's membrane. When the RW membrane is well seen, the surgeon can open it with a little hook. Drilling the cristae fenestrae is a fundamental surgical step to prevent any obstacles to the insertion of rigid arrays.

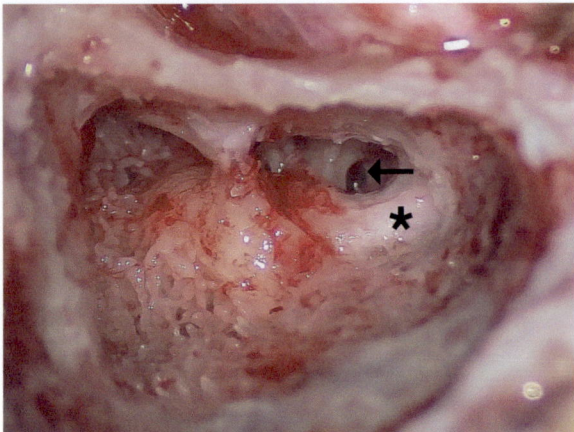

Fig. 2.1 Standard transmastoid approach. Faciale nerve (asterisk), round window (arrow)

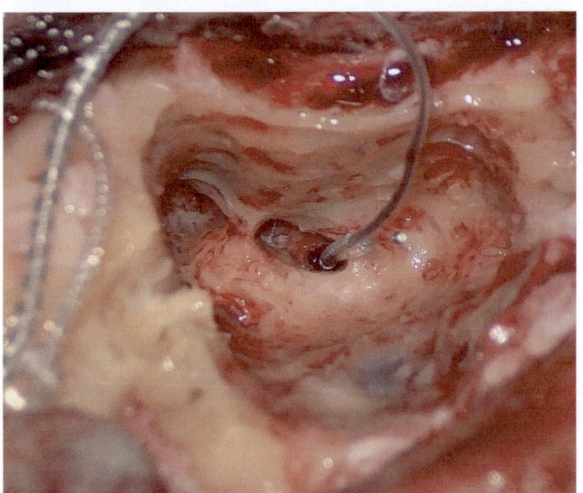

Fig. 2.2 Correct array insertion through a standard approach

2.2 Subtotal Petrosectomy

The subtotal petrosectomy (SP) has been popularized by Hugo Fisch in the 1970s [1] and first applied to the cochlear implant (CI) surgery by Issing [2]. The basic idea is to create a single cavity comprehending the external auditory canal (EAC), the middle ear, and the mastoid. This cavity is completely excluded from the external environment through a blind sac closure of the EAC, packing of the Eustachian tube orifice, and cavity obliteration with fat. Since the original description, a few modification/refinements have been progressively introduced to make the surgery easier and reduce the problems represented by the presence of a foreign body (the CI) [3].

2.2 Subtotal Petrosectomy

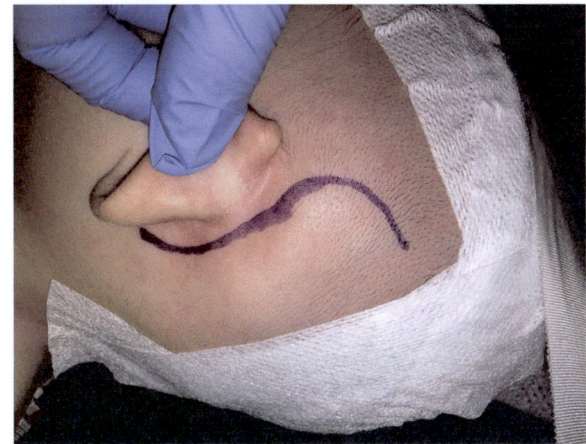

Fig. 2.3 When adapted to the CI surgery, the SP starts with a retroauricolar incision slightly extended postero-superiorly

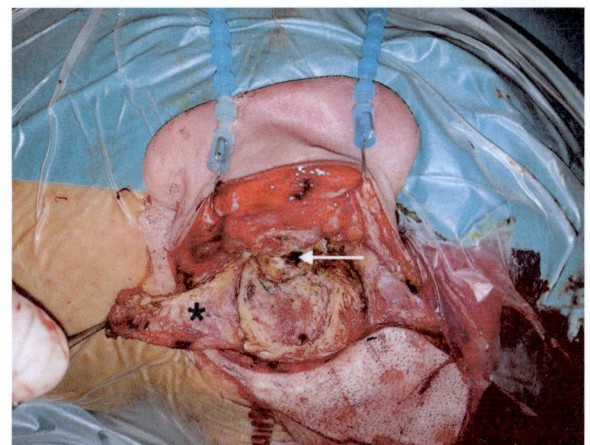

Fig. 2.4 Remaining superficial to the temporalis fascia layer, the EAC (white arrow) is transected for 360°, including the tragal cartilage. An inferiorly based flap (black asterisk) is created from the muscolo-periosteal tissues

First, the retroauricolar skin incision is extended postero-superiorly (Fig. 2.3) in order to accommodate the receiver-stimulator far away from the retroauricolar retraction that often develops after an SP, increasing the risk of an extrusion.

The 360° transection of the EAC is performed more laterally (Fig. 2.4), followed by a two-layer blind-sac closure of the canal itself (Figs. 2.5, 2.6, 2.7, 2.8, 2.9, and 2.10). Meticulous removal of all the EAC medial skin remnants, together with the tympanic membrane (Figs. 2.11, 2.12, 2.13, 2.14, and 2.15), is of utmost importance, since leaving skin behind inevitably leads to cholesteatoma development [4]. A proper canal wall down cavity must be drilled and obtained, with meticulous lowering of the facial ridge and removal/coagulation of the mucosa of the tympanic cavity. All the accessible pneumatized cells of the temporal bone must be removed (Figs. 2.16 and 2.17) and finally the Eustachian tube orifice is packed with muscle/periosteum (Fig. 2.18).

Fig. 2.5 Complete section of the tragal cartilage allows a 180° anterior rotation of the pinna with a more comfortable access to the lateral EAC skin

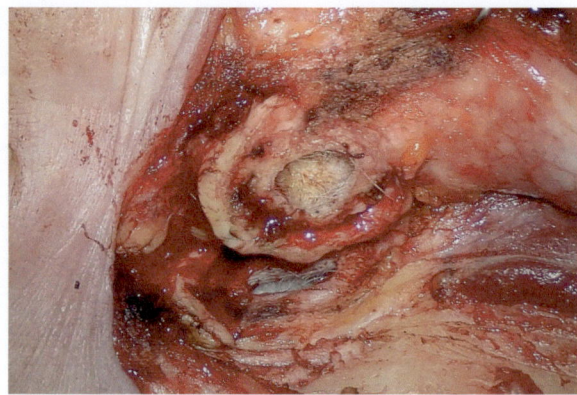

Fig. 2.6 The EAC skin is delicately dissected from the cartilage starting at the level of the tragus

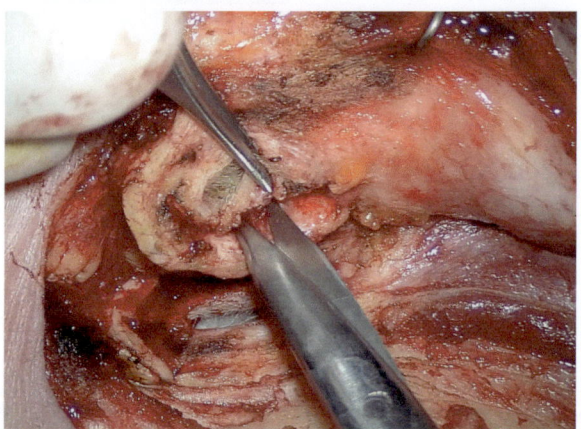

Fig. 2.7 At least 0.5 cm of skin needs to be dissected free for all the 360° of the canal, in order to be easily everted

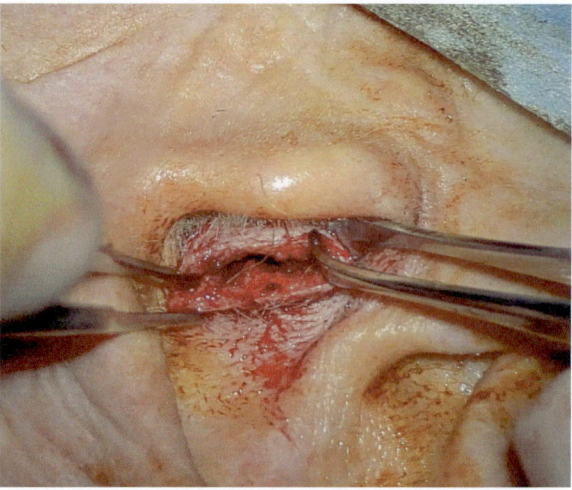

2.2 Subtotal Petrosectomy

Fig. 2.8 The everted skin is sutured; usually 3 or 4 resorbable sutures are sufficient. Cleaning of the area surrounding the suture allows detection of unvoluntary skin tear, potentially causing postoperative complications

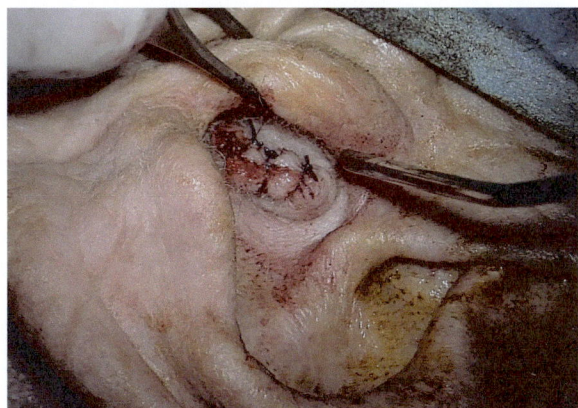

Fig. 2.9 The deep portion of the tragal cartilage is then dissected from the posterior surface of the parotid gland in order to be mobilized

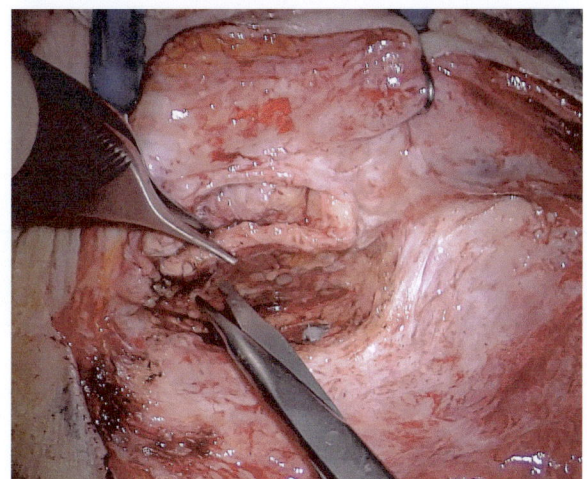

Fig. 2.10 The tragal cartilage is then reflected posteriorly and sutured to the subcutaneous tissues, so representing a strong second layer for the blindsac closure

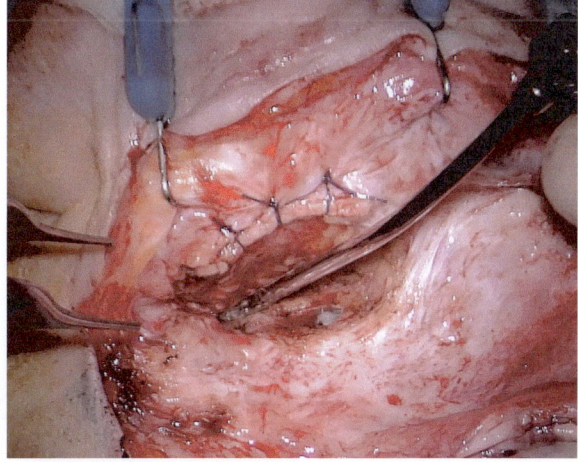

Fig. 2.11 The medial portion of the EAC skin and cartilage are dissected with the electrocautery and a raspatory. The portion of the EAC skin already dissected is then severed as deeper as possible into the canal and removed

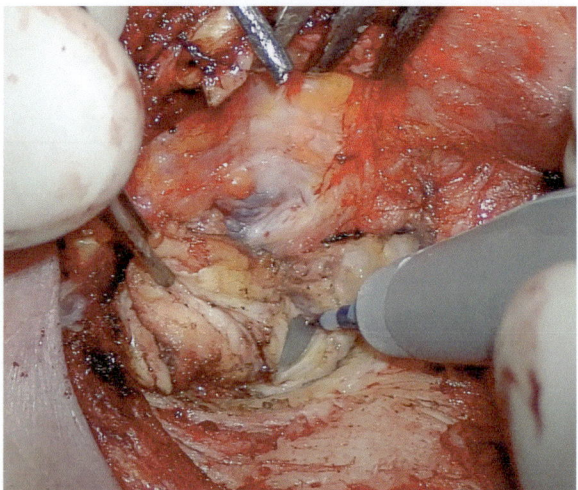

Fig. 2.12 The tympanic membrane, in this case with a perforation, is now clearly on view

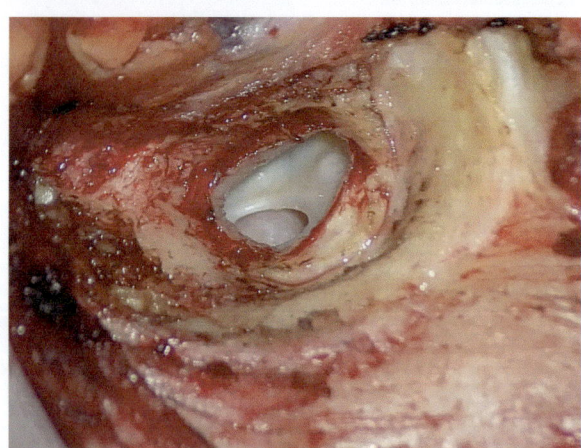

Fig. 2.13 A canal wall-down mastoidectomy is accomplished, including a canalplasty. The posterior anulus is elevated to obtain unobstructed access to the incus (black asterisk)

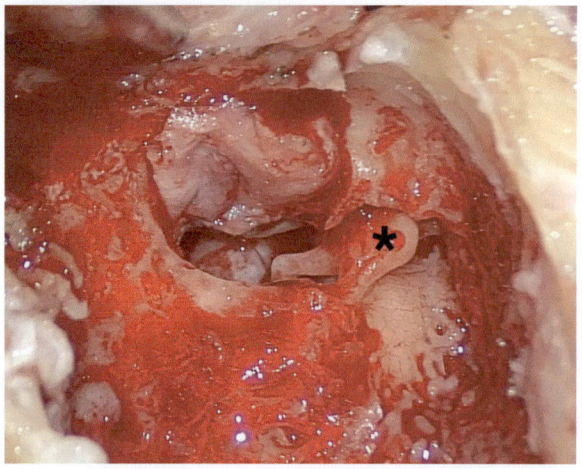

2.2 Subtotal Petrosectomy

Fig. 2.14 Following disarticulation and removal of the incus, the tendon of the tensor tympani is sectioned

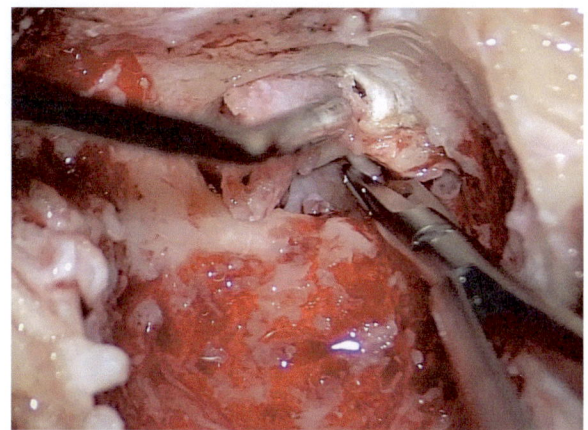

Fig. 2.15 After circumferential dissection of the fibrous anulus, the tympanic membrane is removed en-bloc with the malleus and the remaining portion of the EAC skin

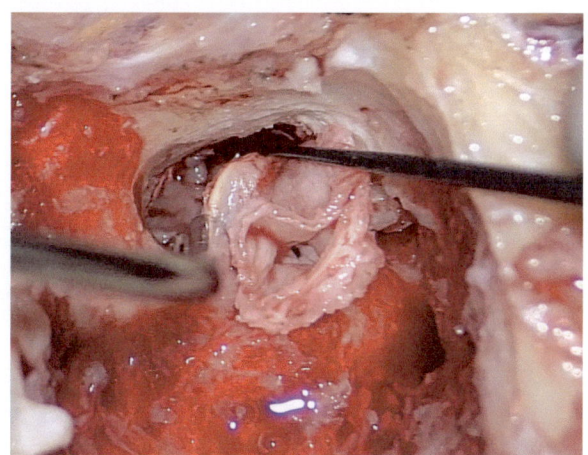

Fig. 2.16 Drilling of the bony anulus is carried on to further reduce the risk to leave some skin remnants. At the same time, the facial ridge is lowered to completely expose the round window (RW) niche

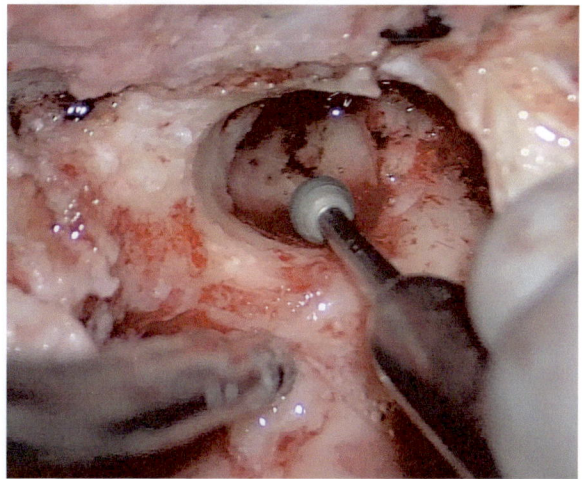

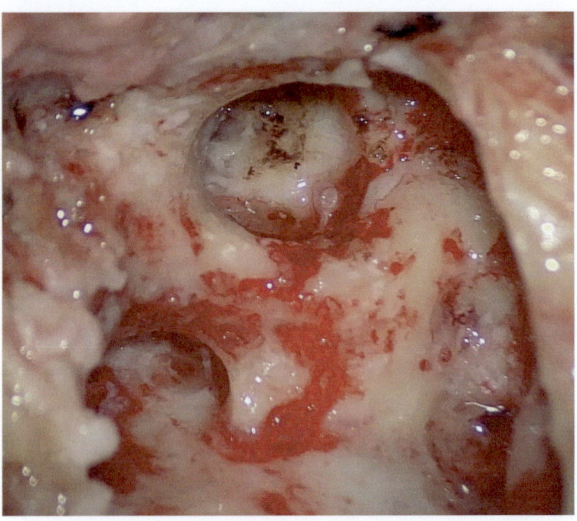

Fig. 2.17 All the accessible pneumatization is drilled away, giving the cavity its final aspect

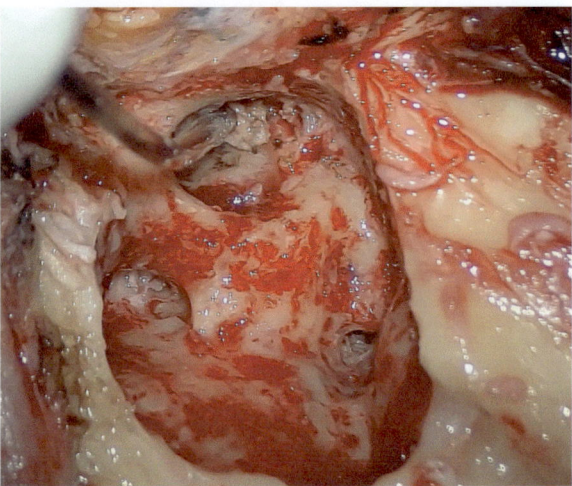

Fig. 2.18 The Eustachian tube orifice is obliterated with muscle and cartilage before positioning of the implant

2.2 Subtotal Petrosectomy

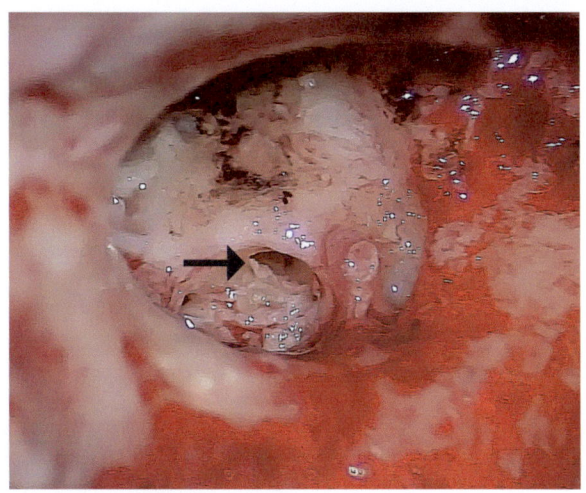

Fig. 2.19 Drilling the anterior and superior border of the round window niche allows the exposure and opening of the Scarpa membrane. In case of use of a rigid array (often required in complex cases), the crista fenestrae (black arrow) is drilled away to facilitate a correct orientation of the insertion

Once a proper view of the RW niche is obtained, the exposure and opening of the membrane are conducted in the standard fashion (Fig. 2.19). While protecting the opened RW, the cradle for the receiver-stimulator must be prepared, paying attention to its position, that should be as much posterior as possible in order to minimize the risk of extrusion (Fig. 2.20). This is also helpful in case an MR is necessary in the follow-up to keep the center of the artifact as far as possible from the anatomical area to be controlled.

The cochlear implantation is carried on by inserting the electrode carrier into the cochlea through the RW (Fig. 2.21). The connecting cable should lay on the medial surface of the cavity, as to reduce the risk of extrusion, and the cavity obliterated with abdominal fat (Figs. 2.22 and 2.23).

Due to the absence of the EAC, it is not possible to close this layer in a watertight fashion. In case a reinforcement is required (mainly in presence of an abundant CSF leak), a temporalis fascia flap may be reflected inferiorly to seal the remaining tissue defect.

Switching from the standard technique to the SP during surgery is even possible; however, it entails a prolongation of the surgical time. [5].

The intraoperative electrophysiological evaluation does not differ from what is commonly executed during a standard cochlear implantation procedure, involving the evaluation of electrodes impedances, the electrodes position, the stapedial reflex evaluation, and finally the EABR.

Fig. 2.20 A cradle is drilled posteriorly and superiorly to the surgical cavity in order to accommodate the receiver-stimulator

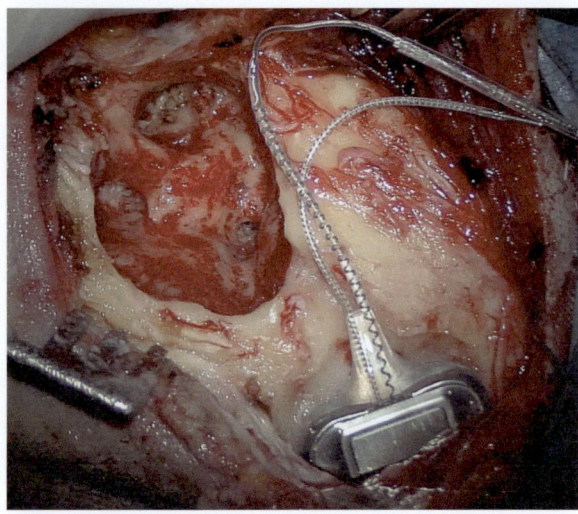

Fig. 2.21 The entire length of the array is slowly inserted in the cochlear lumen. When using an array with a stylet in difficult CI surgery, the stylet is preferentially left in place during the array insertion and removed only at the end of the procedure

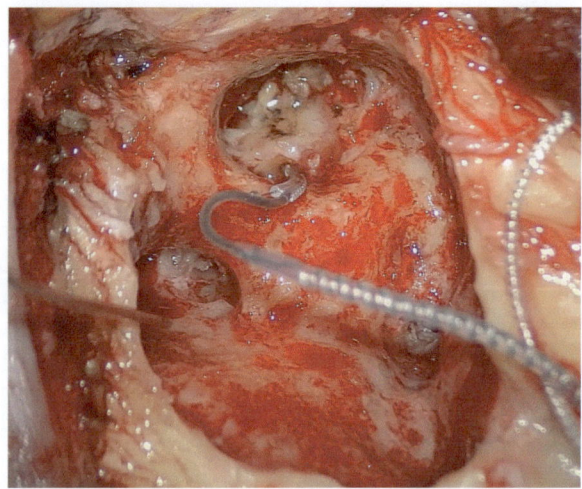

Fig. 2.22 After the standard electrophysiological tests have been completed, the connecting cable is accommodated on the medial wall of the surgical cavity in order to reduce the possibility of extrusion through the retro auricular wound and/or the blind sac closure. The connecting cable is then maintained in place by the fat

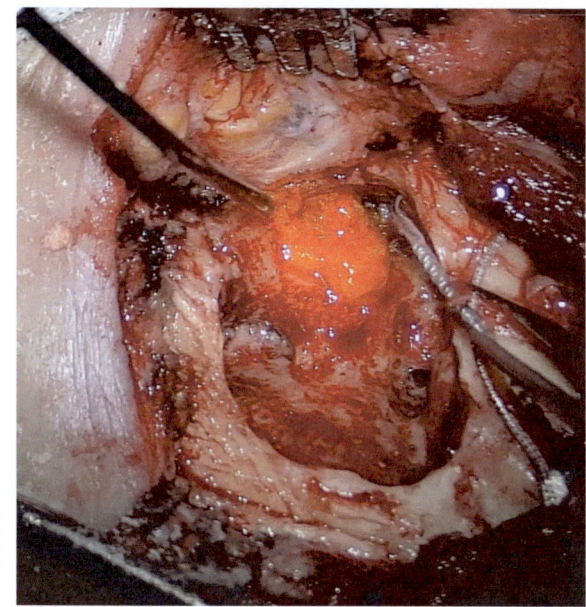

Fig. 2.23 All the surgical cavity is progressively obliterated with abdominal fat

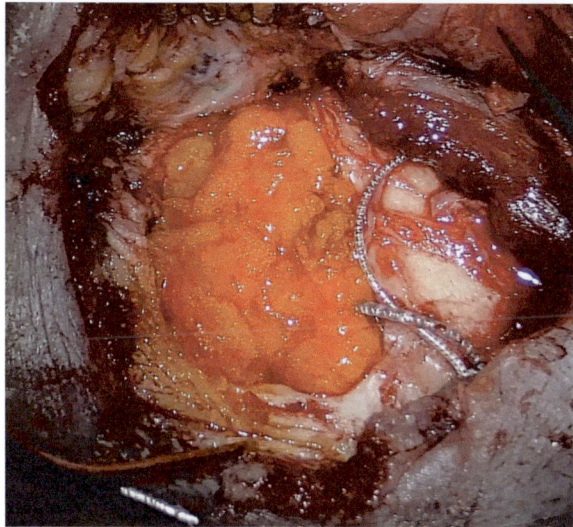

References

1. Coker NJ, Jenkins HA, Fisch U. Obliteration of the middle ear and mastoid cleft in subtotal petrosectomy: indications, technique, and results. Ann Otol Rhinol Laryngol. 1986;95:5.
2. Issing PR, Schonermark MP, Winkelmann S, Kempf HG, Ernst A. Cochlear implantation in patients with chronic otitis: indications for subtotal petrosectomy and obliteration of the middle ear. Skull Base Surg. 1998;8:127–31.
3. D'Angelo G, Donati G, Bacciu A, et al. Subtotal petrosectomy and cochlear implantation. Acta Otorhinolaryngol Ital. 2020;40:450–6. https://doi.org/10.14639/0392-100X-N0931.
4. Pepe G, Franzini S, Guida M, Falcioni M. Subtotal petrosectomy and cochlear implantation: revision surgery. Am J Otolaryngol. 2022;43(3):103333. https://doi.org/10.1016/j.amjoto.2021.103333.
5. Sanna M. Surgery for cochlear and other auditory implants, 2015. Stuttgart: Thieme; 2015.

Preoperative Temporal Bone Imaging in Cochlear Implant Surgery

3

Preoperative radiological study of all cochlear implant (CI) candidates is mandatory [1].

It is usually based on the combination of computed tomography (CT) scan and magnetic resonance imaging (MRI), as the procedures may be seen as complementary, providing different information, fundamental to the likelihood of success of the implantation [2, 3].

MRI scan, with administration of gadolinium and through the study of T1- and T2-weighted images (T1WI and T2WI), according to our institutional routine is performed in adult patients as a screening radiological procedure followed by a preoperative CT scan, while the two procedures are conducted simultaneously in children, under general anesthesia. If the MR study already precludes the possibility of a cochlear implantation, the CT is not performed, representing an exposure of the patient to unnecessary radiation [4].

3.1 Magnetic Resonance Imaging

The study of a preoperative MRI scan in a CI candidate must look for the following features: exclusion of pathologies involving the inner ear, the cerebello-pontine angle (CPA), or the auditory pathway; morphology and patency of the cochlea; morphology of the vestibulo-cochlear nerve and internal auditory canal (IAC); cochlear aperture.

Exclusion of pathologies involving the inner ear, the cerebello-pontine angle (CPA), or the auditory pathway. The presence of a vestibular schwannoma (Fig. 3.1), or other rarer lesions of the CPA such as meningiomas, lipomas, epidermoids, as well as intralabyrinthine schwannomas (Fig. 3.2), must be excluded in CI candidates. Their presence does not automatically exclude the possibility of a CI, but it can jeopardize the result of the procedure and may change the priorities in terms of patient's surgical management [5].

© The Author(s), under exclusive license to Springer Nature Switzerland AG 2025
M. Falcioni et al., *Cochlear Implant - Rare and Difficult Cases*,
https://doi.org/10.1007/978-3-032-02323-0_3

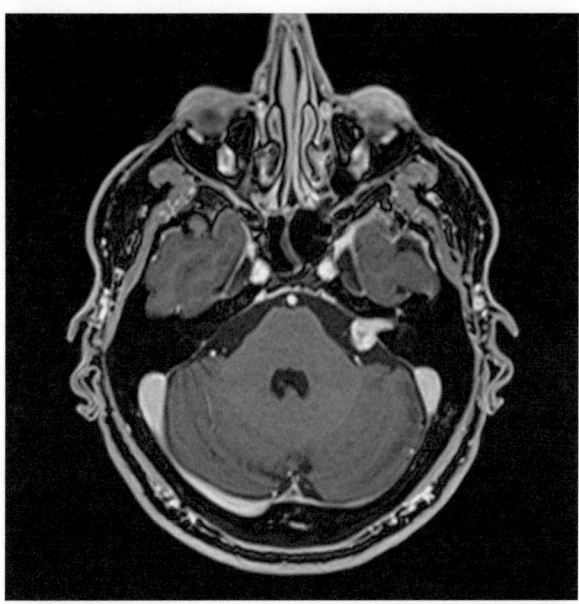

Fig. 3.1 T1WI with gadolinium showing a left vestibular schwannoma

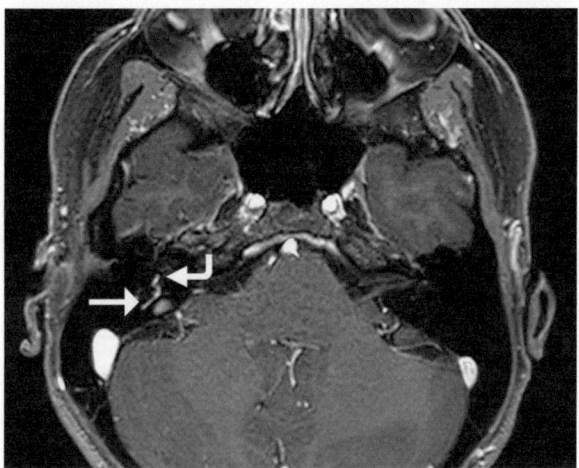

Fig. 3.2 Right-sided labyrinthine schwannoma, involving the vestibule (curved arrow) and the posterior semicircular canal (straight arrow)

Morphology and patency of the cochlea. The importance of MRI scan derives from its capacity of detecting the standard signal of intracochlear fluid in T2 high resolution that allows to confirm the standard anatomy. Even if not absolutely necessary, tridimensional reconstructions allow to obtain a better anatomical representation (Fig. 3.3). Pathological processes associated with sensorineural hearing loss or deafness, as meningitis, labyrinthitis, temporal bone fracture, advanced forms of otosclerosis, may conduce to partial or total membranous labyrinth replacement, changing the standard visualization of the inner ear fluids. In the early stages, this process may be fibrous in nature, thus undetected through conventional CT-scan

3.1 Magnetic Resonance Imaging

Fig. 3.3 3D MR reconstruction of the inner ear on an axial plane

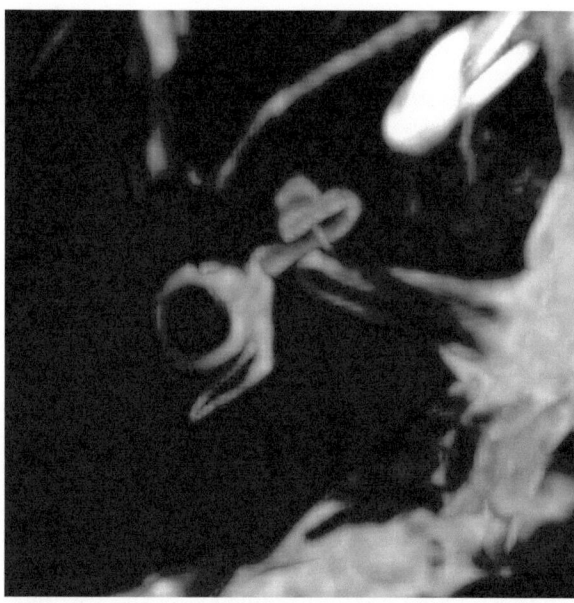

Fig. 3.4 Left-sided inner ear malformation, with the cochlea limited to a small bug (white arrow)

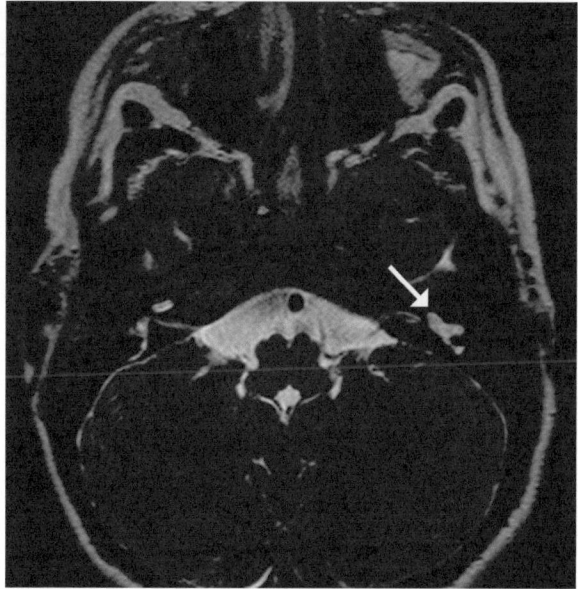

(differently from the ossific phase). Anatomical anomalies of the cochlea (hypoplasia/aplasia, malformations) can also be evaluated (Fig. 3.4) [6].

Anatomical study of the vestibulo-cochlear nerve and internal auditory canal (IAC). Detection of a cochlear nerve hypoplasia is of extreme importance in the

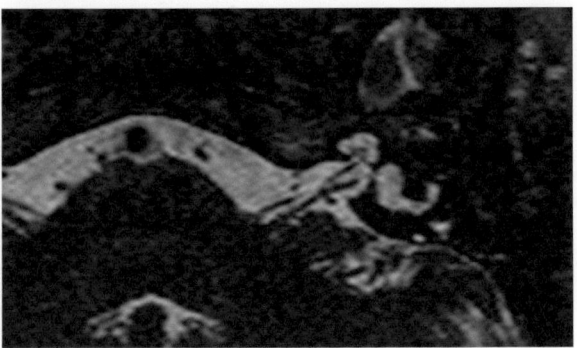

Fig. 3.5 Large cochlear aperture with unobstructed communication between the inner ear and the cerebrospinal fluids

preoperative evaluation, because the resulting performances of a CI are usually reduced when compared with the standard cases. However, from a surgical point of view, cochlear implantation in hypoplasia of the cochlear nerve is performed through a standard surgery. Cochlear nerve aplasia, usually accompanied by the presence of a narrow IAC, must be preoperatively detected with MRI scan, as it represents an absolute contraindication to cochlear implantation. The oblique sagittal T2WI allows a proper evaluation of the IAC fundus and the detection of the former anomalies.

Cochlear aperture. The rare occurrence of a large cochlear aperture (Fig. 3.5) in a normal shaped cochlea must also be investigated, being a probable source of intraoperative cerebrospinal fluid leak.

3.2 Computed Tomography

Once the MRI has excluded any absolute contraindication to the CI surgery, preoperative computed tomography (CT-scan) is the essential radiological study to underline the temporal bone features and it is fundamental for the surgeon to correctly plan the following surgical procedure [7].

Through a high-resolution CT scan, it is possible to identify not only the round window (RW) niche (the final target of the surgery) but also the other important temporal bone structures, the position of which may influence the surgery itself.

As in standard otological surgery, it is mandatory to properly evaluate: the mastoid pneumatization (Fig. 3.6), the position of the middle cranial fossa dura (Fig. 3.7), the sigmoid sinus (SS) (Fig. 3.8), the position of the mastoid facial nerve (FN) (Fig. 3.9), the position of the jugular bulb (JB) (Fig. 3.10), and the internal carotid artery (ICA) (Fig. 3.11). It is mandatory for an otologist to perfectly know the radiological anatomy of temporal bone to recognize any possible anatomical variations and to prevent any surgical risks or damages choosing alternative surgical approaches. CT may even confirm the rare occurrence of a large cochlear aperture (Figs. 3.12 and 3.13) in the contest of a normal shaped cochlea [8].

Fig. 3.6 A sclerotic mastoid has a compact bone and a reduced pneumatization, resulting in a narrower working space. This makes a mastoidectomy and the posterior tympanotomy much more difficult to perform

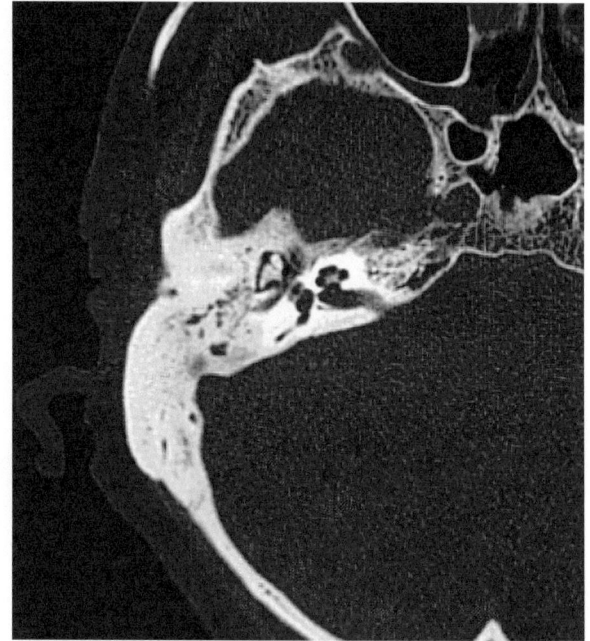

Fig. 3.7 A lower MCF dura (white arrow), in this case running inferiorly to the level of the lateral semicircular canal (black asterisk), can hinder the operative field and obstruct the angle of approach necessary to safely perform a posterior tympanotomy

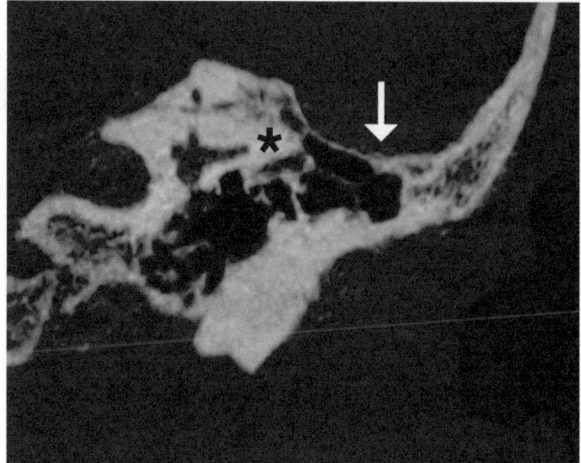

Fig. 3.8 A procident SS (white asterisk) may completely hide and make not accessible the area where to perform the posterior tympanotomy. In this situation, the standard transmastoid approach requires a surgical decompression of the sinus, an unnecessary risky procedure when performing a cochlear implantation

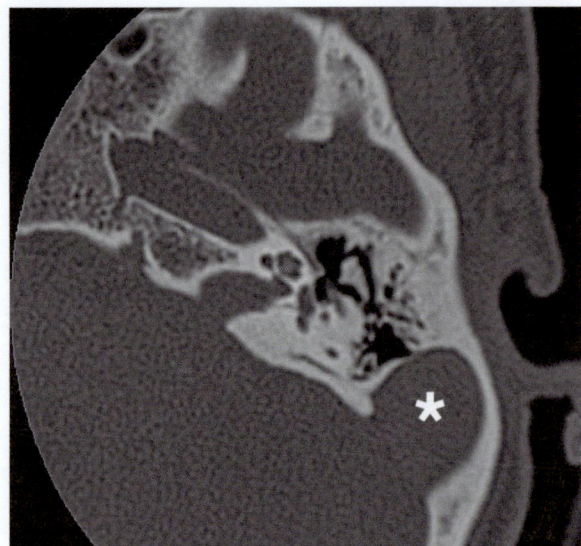

Fig. 3.9 Usually, the third portion of the FN (green arrow) is positioned infero-medially to the lateral semicircular canal (red arrow), without lateral extension beyond this latter

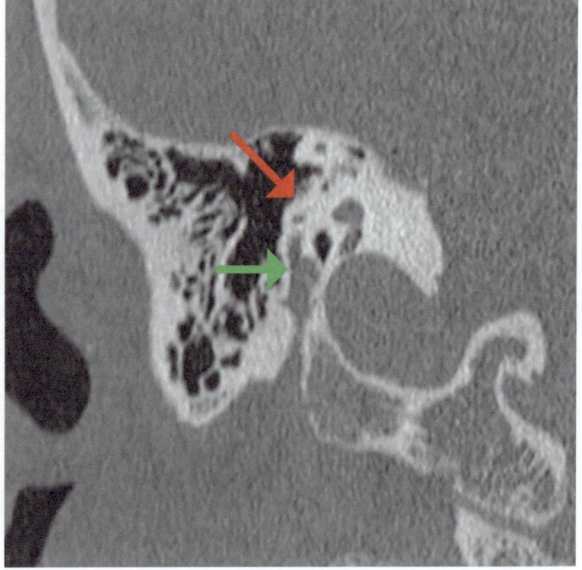

3.2 Computed Tomography

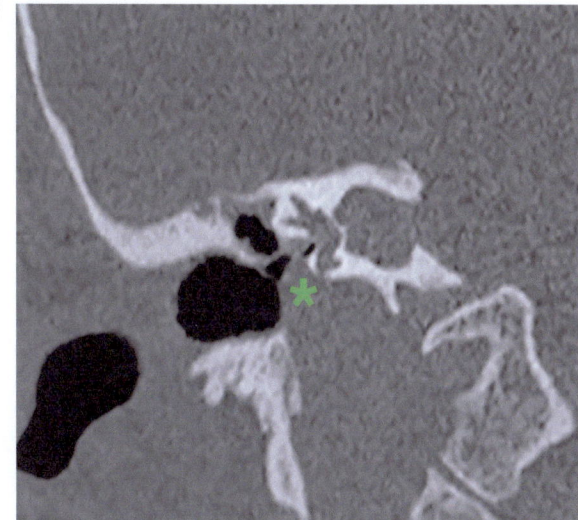

Fig. 3.10 In some situations, a high JB (asterisk) may occupy part of the middle ear cleft, sometime obstructing the RW area. Rarely the dome of the bulb is also without any bony protection, adding additional risk to the surgical maneuvers necessary to reach the RW

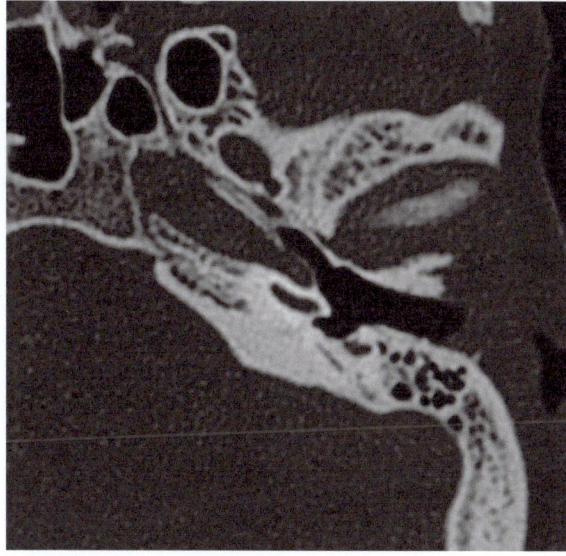

Fig. 3.11 Rare case of lateral extension of the horizontal tract of the carotid artery (see the relationship with the cochlea) still considered in the normal anatomical range

Fig. 3.12 Large cochlear aperture (red arrow)

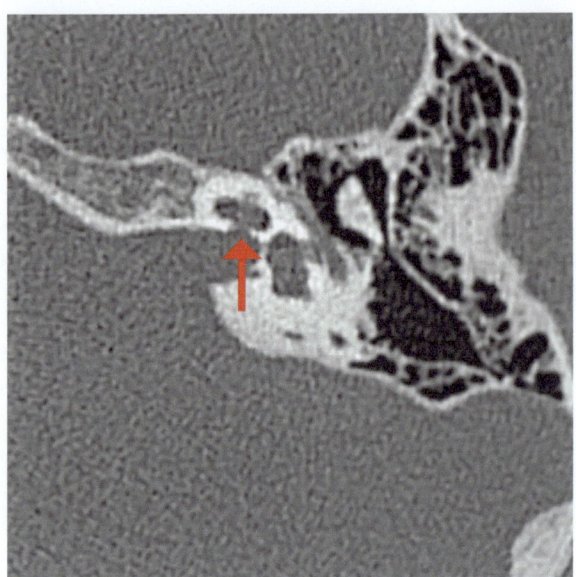

Fig. 3.13 Large cochlear aperture on an inferior plane

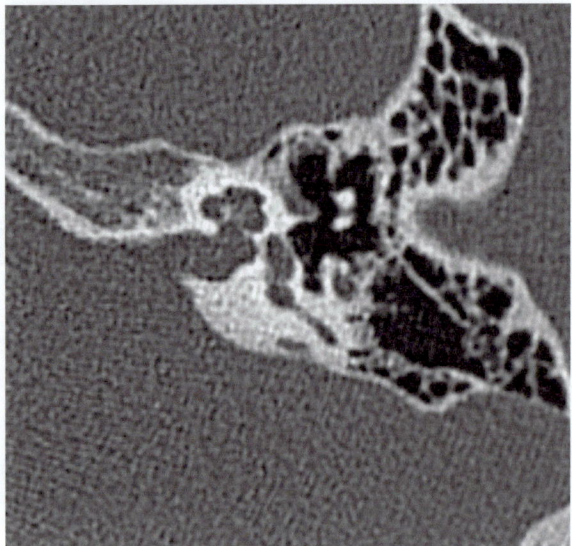

References

1. Swartz JD, Loevner LA. Imaging of the temporal bone. 4th ed. Thieme Medical Publishers, Inc.
2. Sanna M. Surgery for cochlear and other auditory implants, 2015. Stuttgart: Thieme; 2015.
3. Pruitt P. Imaging of the temporal bone DeckerMed Otolaryngol. 2020.
4. Bance M, Zarowski A, Adamson RA, Casselman JW. New imaging modalities in otology. Adv Otorhinolaryngol. 2018;81:1–13.
5. Krainik A, Casselman JW. Imaging evaluation of patients with cranial nerve disorders. IDKD Springer Series [Internet]. 2020:143–61.
6. Silver RD, Djalilian HR, Levine SC, Rimell FL. High-resolution magnetic resonance imaging of human cochlea. Laryngoscope. 2002;112(10):1737–41.
7. Waldeck S, Schmidt S, von Falck C, Chapot R, Brockmann M, Overhoff D. New hybrid multiplanar cone beam computed tomography-laser-fluoroscopic-guided approach in cochlear implant surgery. Int J Comp Assist Radiol Surg. 2022;17(10):1837–43.
8. Cornwall HL, Marway PS, Bance M. A micro-computed tomography study of round window anatomy and implications for atraumatic cochlear implant insertion. Otology Neurotol. 2020;42(2):327–34.

Variations of the Temporal Bone Anatomy with Surgical Implication for Cochlear Implant Surgery

4

When performing a cochlear implantation, the possibility of encountering an anatomical variation must be always considered, especially in the pediatric population. Some anatomical variations may represent an obstacle or a challenge, indeed [1]. Those variations most commonly found (as in standard otological surgery) are as follows: an high jugular bulb (JB) that can obstacle the round window (RW) niche access (Figs. 4.1, 4.2, 4.3, 4.4, 4.5, 4.11, 4.13, 4.14, 4.15, 4.16, 4.17, and 4.18), an anteriorly positioned sigmoid sinus (SS) (Figs. 4.10, 4.12, and 4.19), the presence of a low middle cranial fossa (MCF) dura, a lateral mastoid portion of the facial nerve (Figs. 4.6, 4.7, 4.8, and 4.9), or a poorly pneumatized mastoid [2]. In rare situations, the all mastoids may be inaccessible, requiring a transcanal approach (Figs. 4.20, 4.21, 4.22, 4.23, 4.24, and 4.25). The preoperative selection of the surgical approach must be based on a proper radiological study, as described in Chap. 3.

Nevertheless, sometimes the type of anatomical variation and the difficulty that may derive from make the selection of a subtotal petrosectomy (SP) mandatory [3]; in other situations, the standard transmasotid approach could be riskier but still feasible. Some clinical cases of anatomical variation are illustrated and discussed [4, 5].

Case 4.1 High jugular bulb

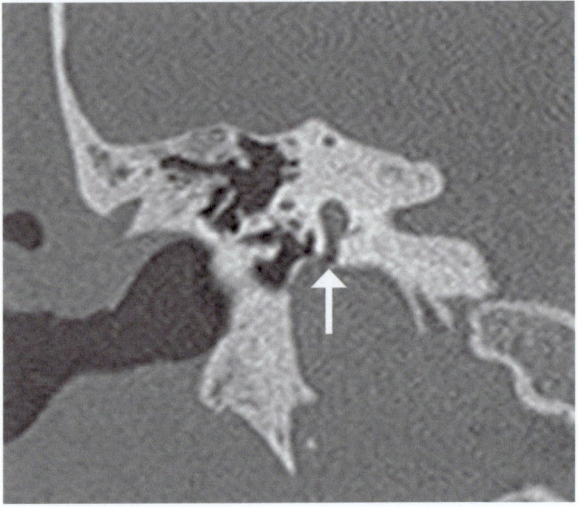

Fig. 4.1 Preoperative CT scan, coronal view. The JB is high and completely hides the RW niche (white arrow). The vessel is covered by a thin bone layer

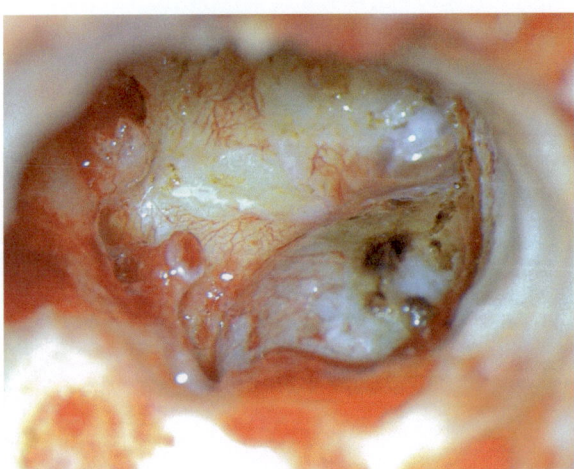

Fig. 4.2 A subtotal petrosectomy is performed to have a better access to the promontorium and perform a cochleostomy. The RW niche is completely obstructed by the JB dome. Surgical decompression of the bulb, even if technically feasible, is a procedure with a high risk of bleeding or thrombosis. The SP guarantees space and brightness enough to expose safely the JB and to drill out the cochlea. In addition, any possible intraoperative complication is better managed through the SP

Fig. 4.3 After drilling the promontorium immediately anterior to the JB (white asterisk), the endostium of the cochlea (black asterisk) is identified

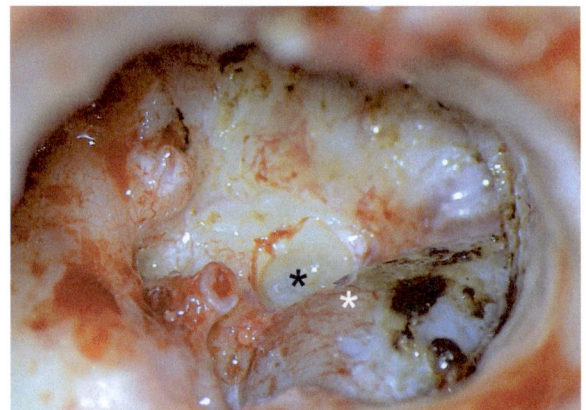

Fig. 4.4 Opening of the basal turn of the cochlea, with exposure of scala tympani (white asterisk) and scala vestibuli (black asterisk)

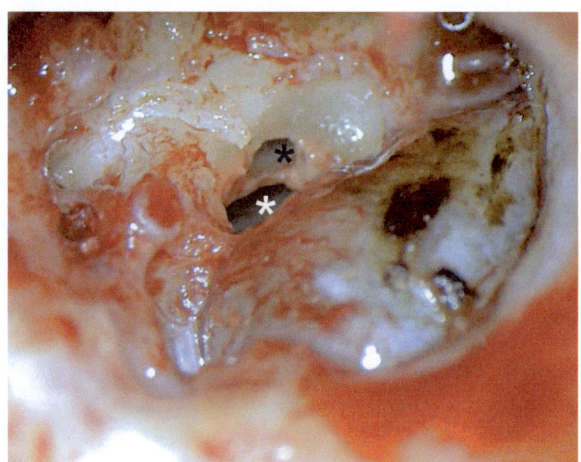

Fig. 4.5 Total insertion of the array into scala tympani; the basilar membrane, pushed superiorly by the array, is clearly visible

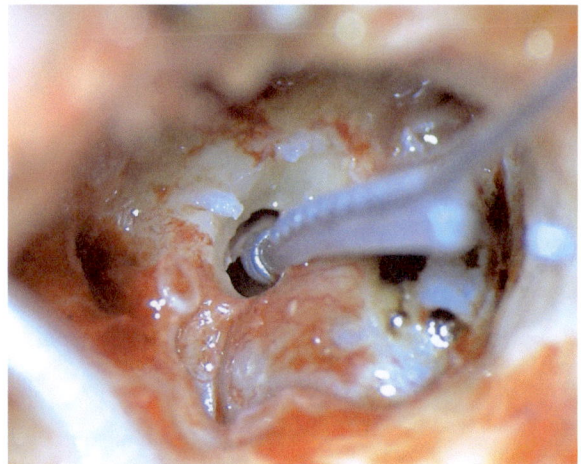

Case 4.2 Lateral and anterior route of the FN

Fig. 4.6 A lateral route of the mastoid portion of the FN, running lateral to the dome of the lateral semicircular canal, is radiologically identified on the coronal section of the preoperative CT. Compare with standard situation on Fig. 3.9

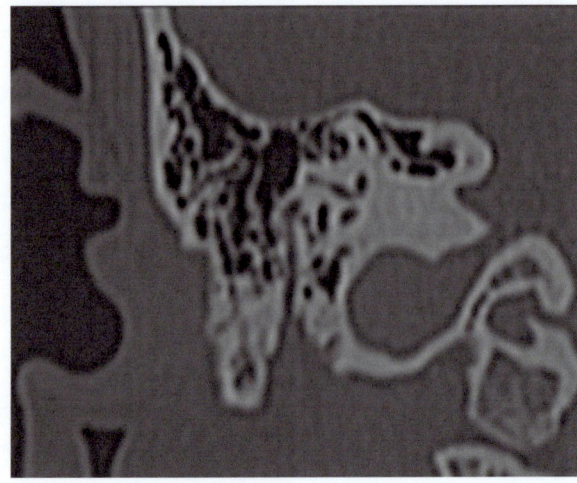

Fig. 4.7 During surgery (standard approach), the nerve (black asterisk) was identified in a lateral and anterior position respect to the LSC (white asterisk). Consequently, the room available for the posterior tympanotomy was narrowed

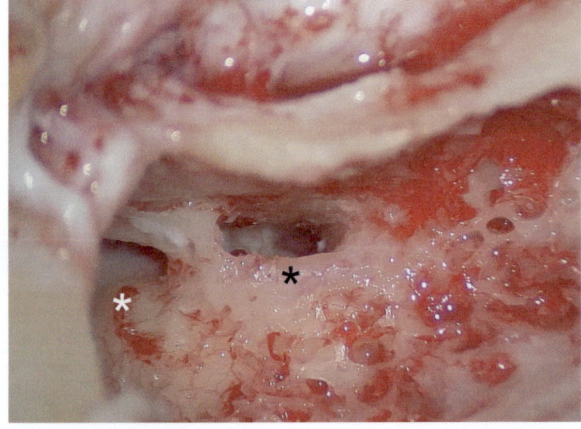

Fig. 4.8 Despite the narrow approach, the RW is correctly exposed

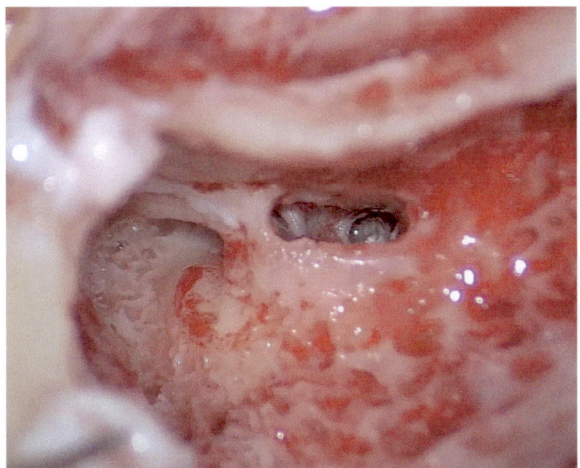

Fig. 4.9 Total insertion of the array is achieved

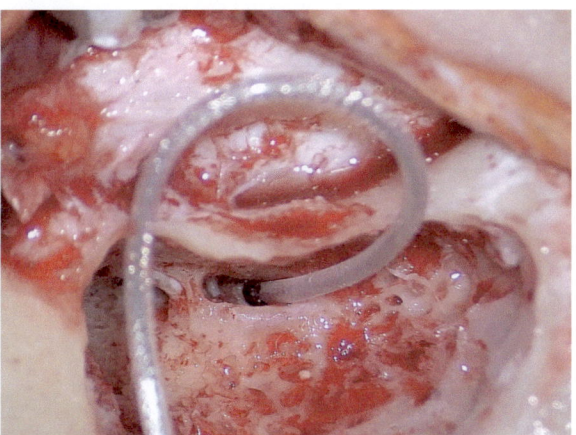

Case 4.3 *Procident sigmoid sinus and high jugular bulb*

Fig. 4.10 Axial preoperative CT scan showing procident right SS (white asterisk), almost reaching the posterior wall of the external auditory canal. The surgical option of the SP is consequently selected

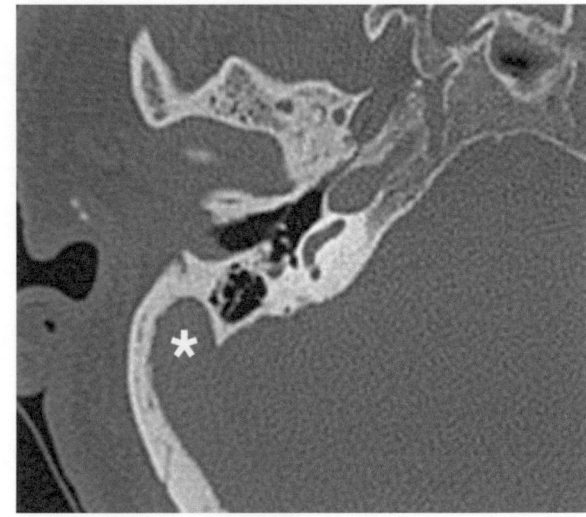

Fig. 4.11 Coronal preoperative CT scan showing a high JB, covered by a thick bony wall, reaching the RW niche

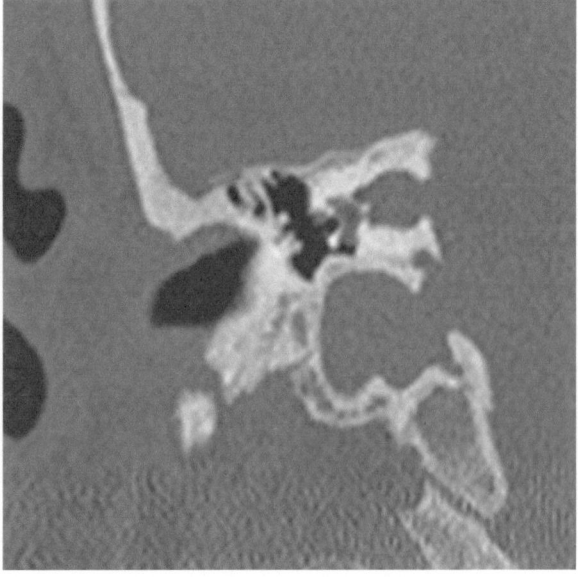

Fig. 4.12 Drilling of cortical layer of mastoid bone immediately exposes the procident SS (white asterisk) confirming its proximity to the posterior wall of the external auditory canal

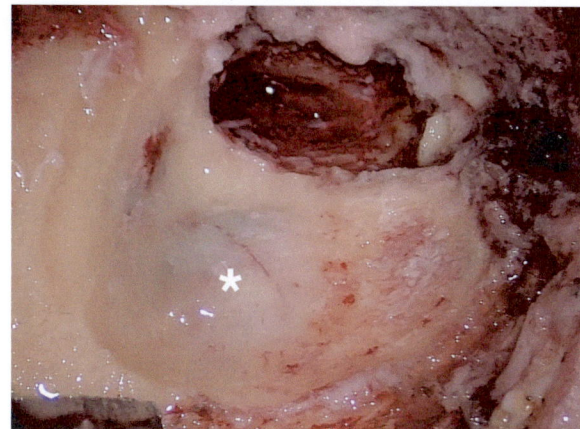

Fig. 4.13 After the SP has been completed, the RW (black arrow) is only partially visible because of the high JB (black asterisk)

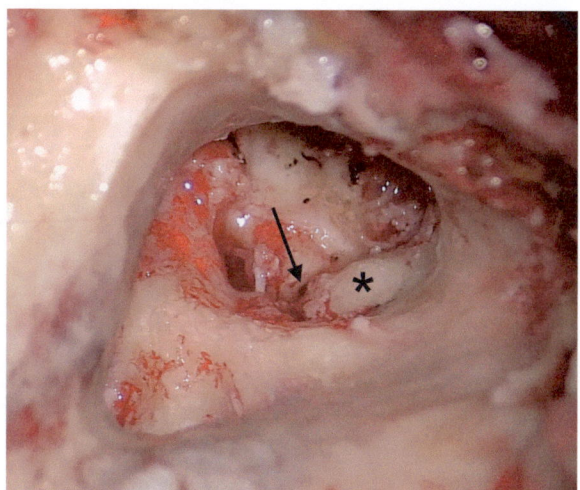

Fig. 4.14 The bony dome of the JB is gently drilled with a diamond burr to expose the RW

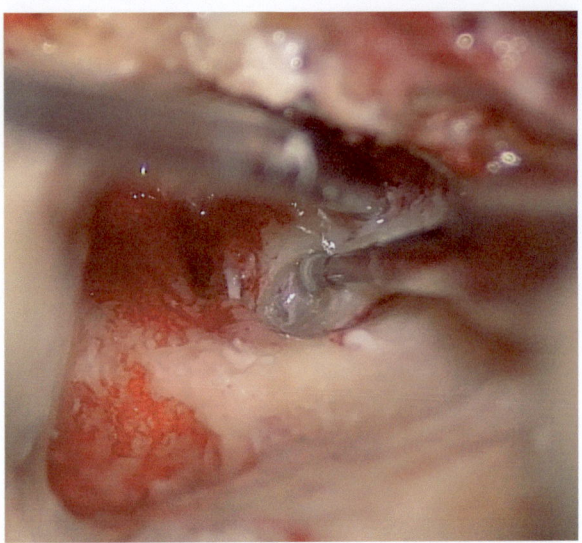

Fig. 4.15 The JB surface is still not visible for transparency, but thinning of the bony dome has allowed a sufficient exposure of the RW niche (white arrow)

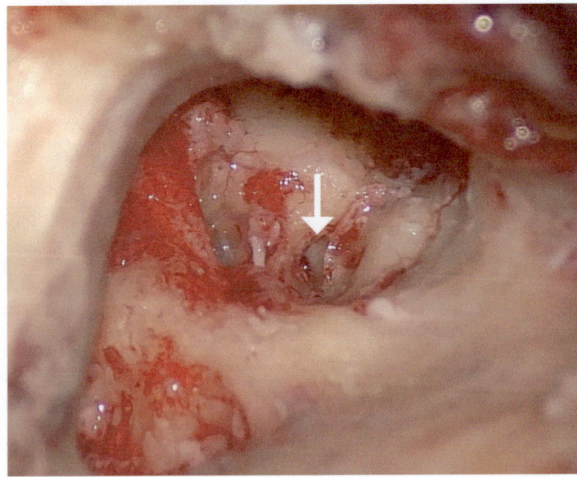

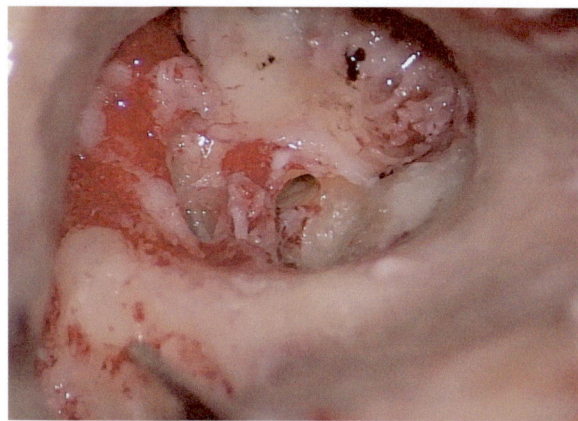

Fig. 4.16 The RW membrane is opened and the cochlear lumen exposed

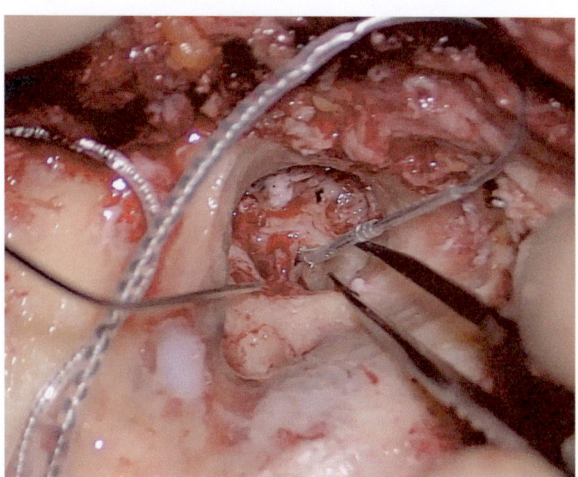

Fig. 4.17 The array is easily introduced into the cochlear lumen

Fig. 4.18 Obliteration of the RW with abdominal fat

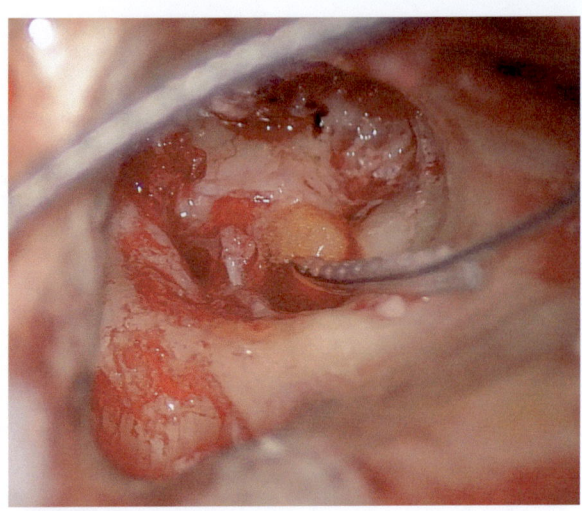

Fig. 4.19 Post-op CT scan, axial view, showing the array correctly in place and the skeletonization of the SS

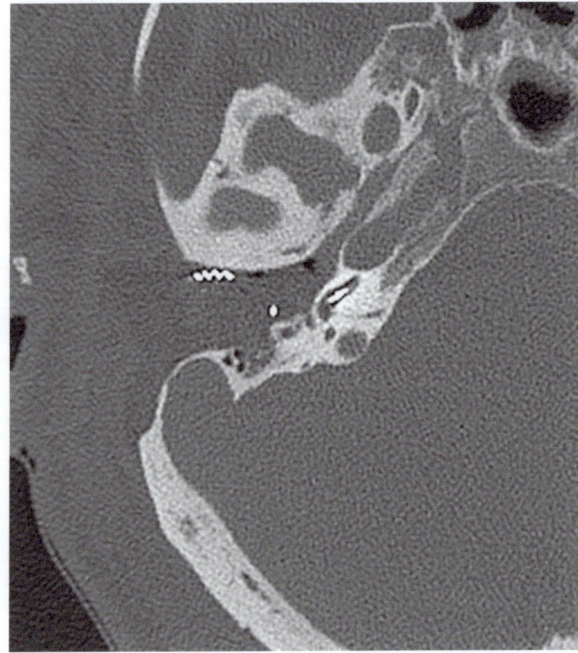

4 Variations of the Temporal Bone Anatomy with Surgical Implication for Cochlear... 37

Case 4.4 *Vascular malformation of the mastoid, making impossible any transmastoid route, combined with a high jugular bulb and a persistent stapedial artery. A large canalplasty with blindsac occlusion of the EAC has been considered the only available option.*

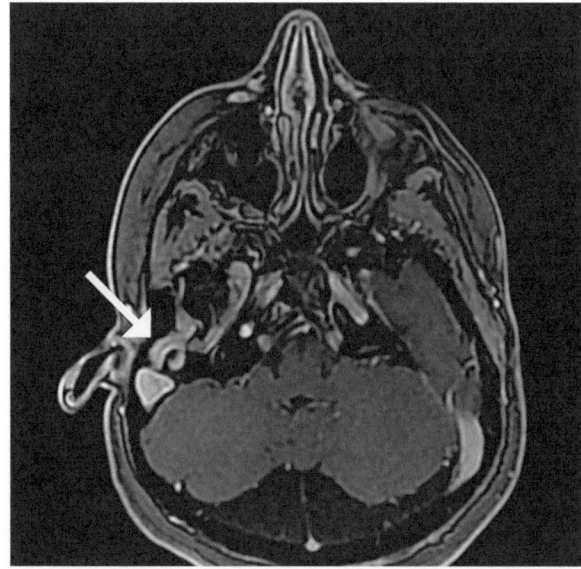

Fig. 4.20 Axial MR showing a large venous vessel (white arrow) crossing the mastoid, with no room available for a mastoidectomy

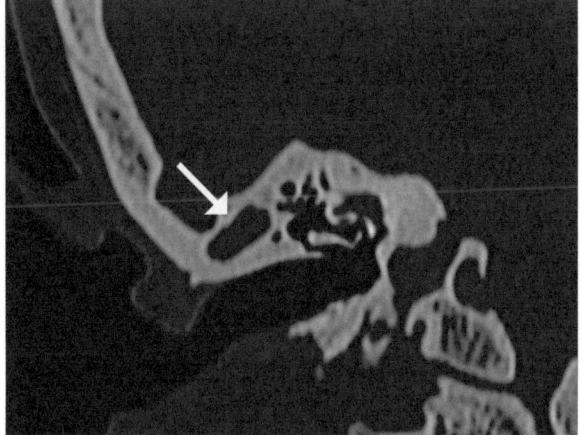

Fig. 4.21 Coronal TC confirming the inaccessibility of the mastoid due to the large vein (white arrow). The jugular bulb is very close to the round window too

Fig. 4.22 After removing the tympanic membrane, the malleus, and the incus, the EAC is enlarged as much as possible to gain access to the middle ear cleft. The RW niche (black arrow) appears as a thin fissure due to the high jugular bulb (black asterisk). Superiorly to the RW, a persistent stapedial artery (white asterisk) is also visible

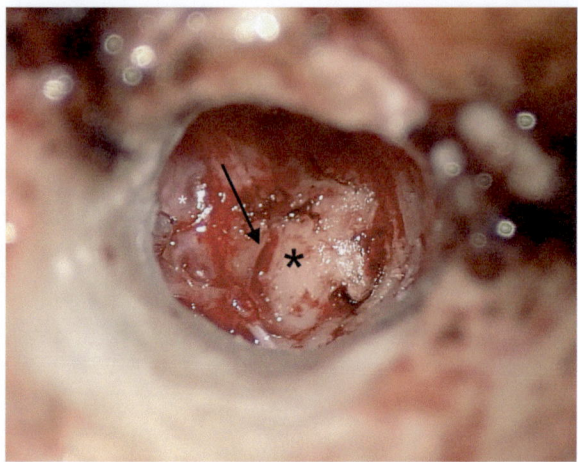

Fig. 4.23 Delicate drilling of the bone on top of the jugular bulb allows exposure of the RW (black arrow)

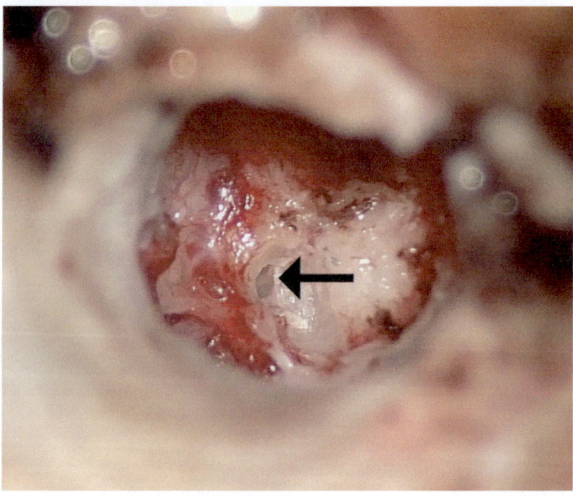

Fig. 4.24 The RW is completely opened to allow easy access to the scala tympany even if through the unfavorable angle offered by the trans-canal approach. The persistent stapedial artery (white asterisk) is clearly visible running in between the stapes crura

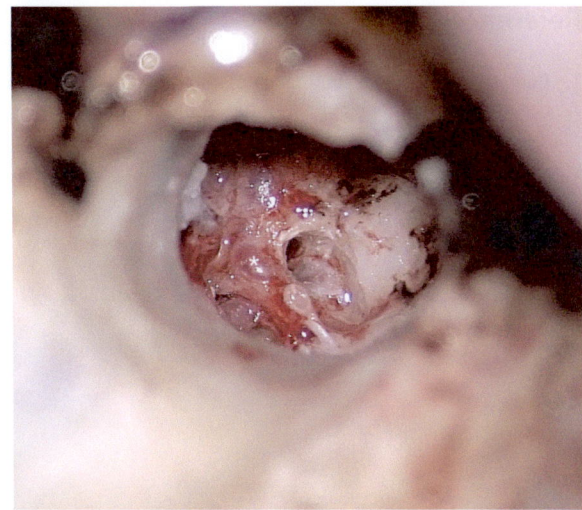

Fig. 4.25 The array is finally inserted into the cochlear lumen

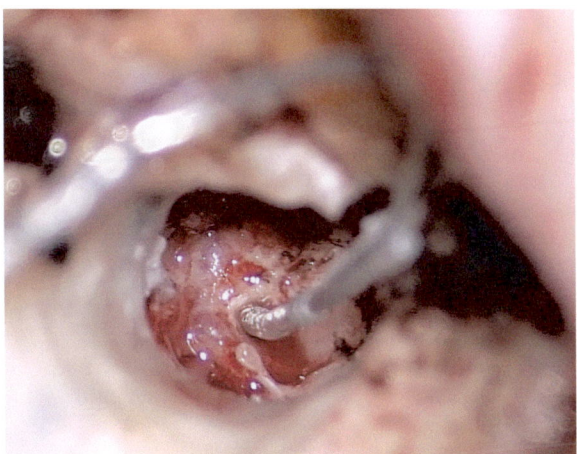

References

1. Issing PR, et al. Cochlear implantation in patients with chronic otitis: Indications for subtotal petrosectomy and obliteration of the Middle Ear. Skull Base. 1998;8(03):127–31. https://doi.org/10.1055/s-2008-1058571.
2. D'Angelo G, et al. Subtotal petrosectomy and cochlear implantation. Acta Otorhinolaryngologica Italica. 2020;40(6):450–6. https://doi.org/10.14639/0392-100x-n0931.
3. Sanna M. Surgery for cochlear and other auditory implants, 2015. Stuttgart: Thieme; 2015.
4. Swartz JD, Loevner LA. Imaging of the temporal bone. 4th ed. Thieme Medical Publishers, Inc.
5. Pepe G, Franzini S, Guida M, Falcioni M. Subtotal petrosectomy and cochlear implantation: revision surgery. Am J Otolaryngol. 2022;43(3):103333. https://doi.org/10.1016/j.amjoto.2021.103333.

Cochlear Implantation in Advanced Otosclerosis

5

Cochlear implantation in otosclerosis is the auditory rehabilitation modality of choice for cases with severe to profound sensorineural hearing losses that cannot be managed with conventional surgery or hearing aids (advanced otosclerosis) [1].

In the majority of the patients, a piston positioned during a previous surgery (Fig. 5.2) is found in place of the stapes suprastructure, but this does not entail any additional surgical difficulty. The main challenge arising in implanting patients with advanced forms of otosclerosis derives from the cochlear modifications, especially from the degree of ossification (Figs. 5.1, 5.11, and 5.12); these latter may be associated with a partial insertion of the electrode array or array dislocation from the scala tympani to the scala vestibuli. In severe cases of advanced otosclerosis, the risk of CSF leakage during surgery must be considered [2], as well as postoperative facial nerve stimulation. Furthermore, patients with advanced otosclerosis may manifest cavitary changes surrounding the cochlea (Figs. 5.24 and 5.25), sometimes reaching the internal auditory canal [3]. In cavitating cases, extracochlear insertion represents the most dangerous complication of surgery, due to the false lumen created by the osseous rearrangement (Figs. 5.25, 5.26, 5.27, 5.28, 5.29, and 5.30).

As for standard cochlear implants candidates, also in otosclerosis the preoperative imaging study plays a pivotal role. Computed tomography scan (CT-scan) and magnetic resonance imaging (MRI) are required and must be meticulously studied as to determine the degree of ossification and/or the cavitary bony changes.

The evaluation of the degree of cochlear ossification in advanced otosclerosis is usually accomplished through CT scan of the temporal bone. According to Rotteveel et al. [4], the ossification range may vary from the initial and isolated involvement of the round window (RW) niche (solely fenestral lesion—type 1) to the involvement of the whole cochlea (severe retrofenestral lesion—type 3) with loss of its normal aspect, passing through middle stages (type 2) of retrofenestral ossification, with or without fenestral involvement. Additional CT findings include the double-ring effect and the narrowed basal turn [5]. Schematically, this classification traduces into practice since it helps in defining the most appropriate surgical strategy:

standard CI with posterior tympanotomy and RW approach seems to be reasonable in ossification limited to the fenestral area. In cases of mild basal turn involvement, it is up to surgeon's preference and experience, while in type 3 and in cavitary forms, SP is strongly advised [6]. However, in some cases, the CT images may overestimate the effective degree of involvement; cochleae with a completely subverted anatomy on CT have been successfully implanted.

In every case in which, due to the grade of cochlear ossification, there is the risk of incomplete electrode insertion or its misplacement, a SP must be planned, or the surgeon should be able to switch to it during surgery with no hesitation whenever difficulties are encountered. SP offers a better view and access to the surgical field, also allowing the surgeon to execute wide cochlear drill-out looking for a cochlear lumen (Figs. 5.3, 5.4, 5.5, 5.6, 5.7, 5.8, 5.13, 5.14, 5.15, 5.16, 5.17, 5.18, 5.19, and 5.20) [7, 8].

After having been able to identify a cochlear lumen, the insertion of a depth gauge is strongly suggested. The use of a short and rigid electrode, preferably with a stylet, is advised, avoiding atraumatic arrays with higher chances to bend when introduced in a not completely free cochlear lumen. When adopting an array with a stylet, it is better to achieve the full introduction before removing the stylet. Scala vestibuli insertion may represent an alternative option in severe ossification involving mainly the scala tympani. As for the majority of standard cochlear implants, also in otosclerosis patient, correct positioning of the array is postoperatively checked with a CT scan (Figs. 5.8, 5.20, and 5.31).

Even implant activation and mapping (Figs. 5.9, 5.10, 5.21, 5.22, 5.23, 5.32, 5.33, and 5.34) in otosclerosis cases may represent a challenge. As already mentioned, facial nerve stimulation represents one possible complications of cochlear implantation (CI) in otosclerosis patients, because the diffusion of the electric stimulation is different in the otoslerotic bone. Intraoperative electrophysiological testing is crucial to evaluate those stimulation levels that can interfere with facial nerve function; this can be of huge help postoperatively in selecting the proper cochlear nerve stimulation during the mapping process.

In patients presenting facial nerve stimulation following CI activation, some strategies may be adopted by the audiologist to overcome the problem: changing the ratio of electrical stimulation, reducing the rate of stimulation per-each electrode, or, in complex cases usually with severe grade of cochlear ossification, changing the entire stimulation modality (bipolar, bipolar +1, or pseudomonopolar). The latter strategies are able to generate intracochlear stimulation arches, limiting the electrical stimuli diffusion and consequently facial nerve stimulation.

Another possible strategy to reduce/resolve facial nerve stimulation is to identify and deactivate the cochlear implant electrodes close to the perigeniculate area (frequently those located in the middle/apical turns, the closest to the route of the nerve), always bearing in mind that a maximum of three to four electrodes can be switched off without reduction of the patient hearing performance.

Electrode array translocation from the tympanic to the vestibular scala or the opposite creates a trauma with fibrosis that may require an increase in the stimulation levels (case number 5.2) (Fig. 5.21, 5.22, and 5.23).

Implanted patients with otosclerosis must be properly followed up as to detect any worsening of the hearing performance. This is generally related to the possible progression of cochlear ossification even after the cochlear implantation.

5 Cochlear Implantation in Advanced Otosclerosis

Case 5.1 *Left sided otosclerosis with ossification: subtotal petrosectomy with scala tympani insertion*

Fig. 5.1 Reconstructed CT images along the cochlear planes allow a better understanding of the ossification extension (white arrow)

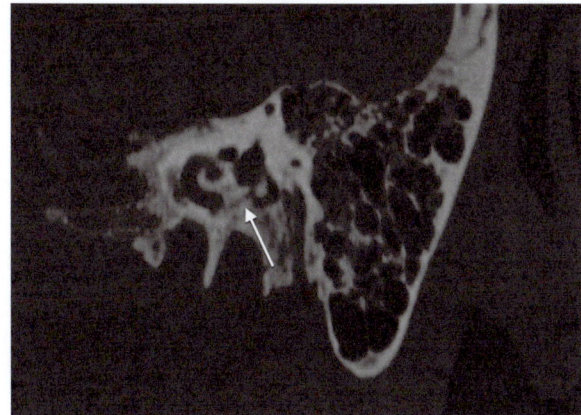

Fig. 5.2 SP; section of the piston inserted during previous stapedotomy (a common finding in otosclerosis cases)

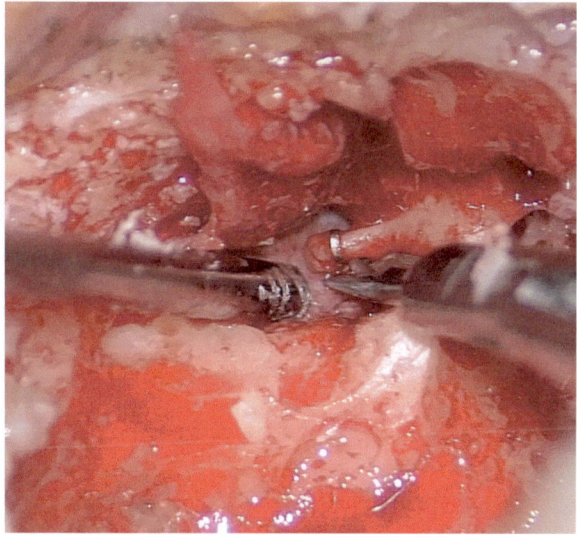

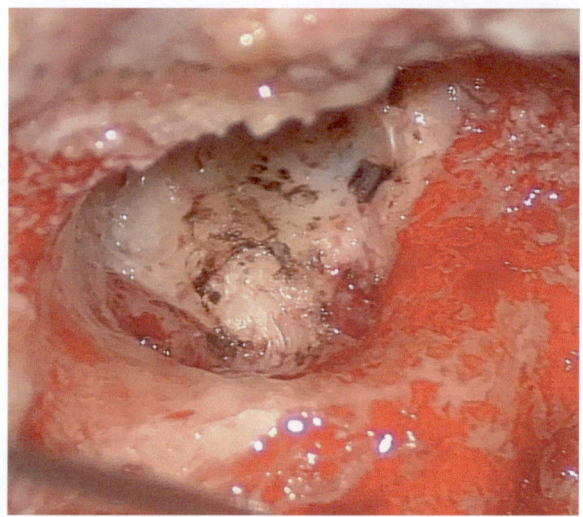

Fig. 5.3 Appearance of the surgical field after completion of the SP. Note the difficulties in identifications of the windows

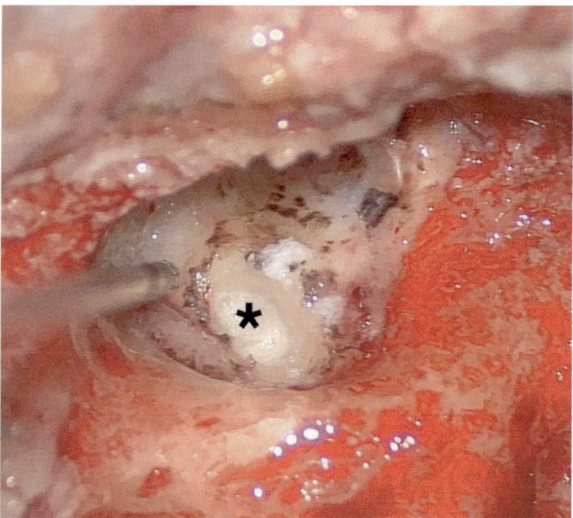

Fig. 5.4 After the initial promontorium drilling (black asterisk), there is still no evidence of the cochlear lumen

Fig. 5.5 Further anterior extension of the drilling allows opening of the cochlear lumen (white arrow), probably the scala vestibuli

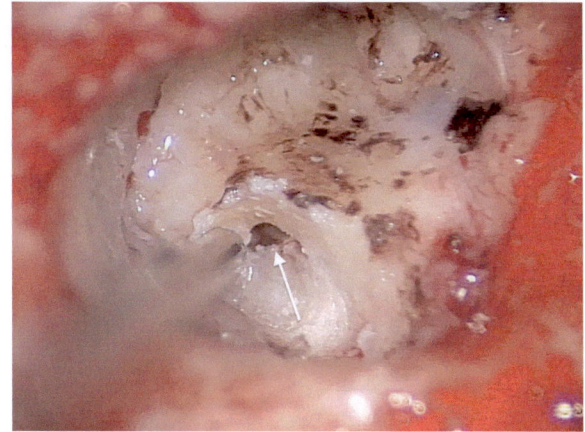

Fig. 5.6 Both the scala tympani (white asterisk) and the scala vestibuli (green asterisk) are now clearly in view

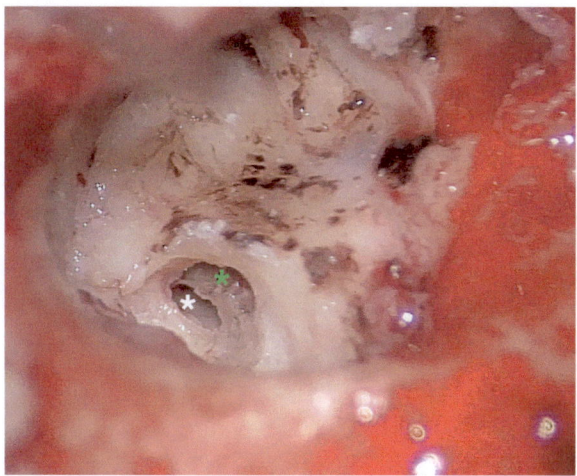

Fig. 5.7 The array is progressively pushed in the scala tympani

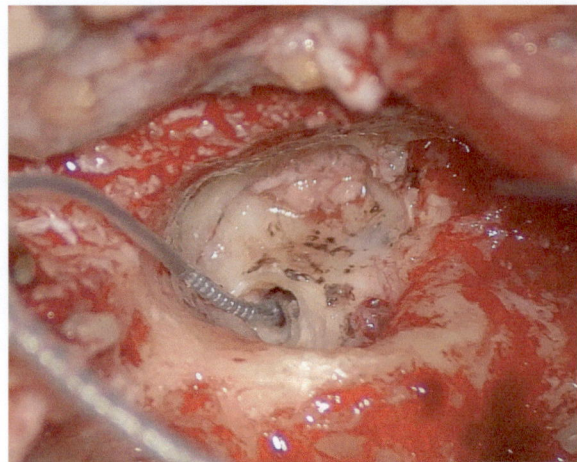

Fig. 5.8 Postoperative CT showing the complete array insertion in the contest of an SP

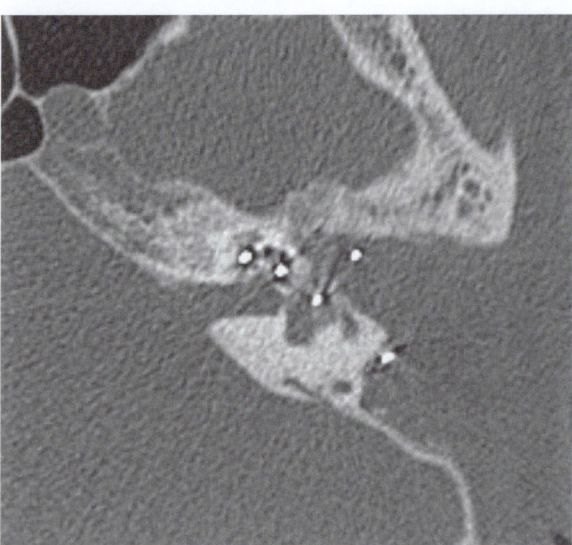

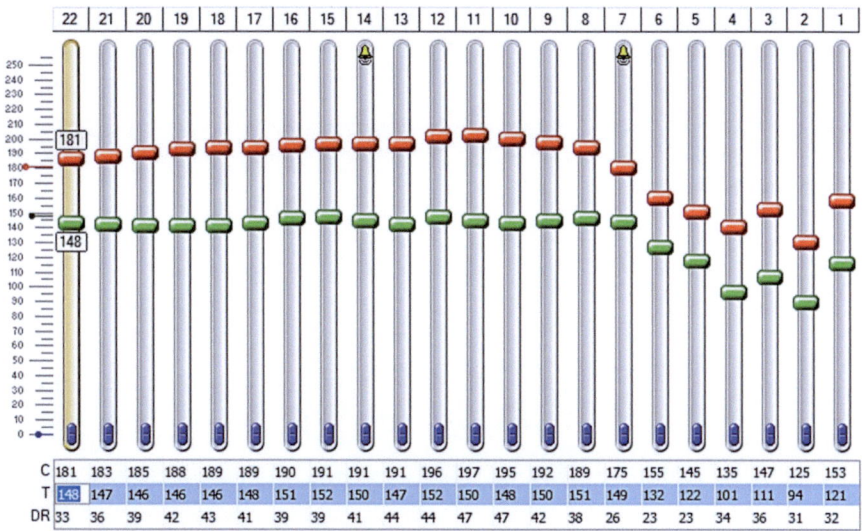

Fig. 5.9 Due to otosclerotic process, stimulation levels in the middle and apical turns are higher than in the basal turn, even if this latter has been partially drilled

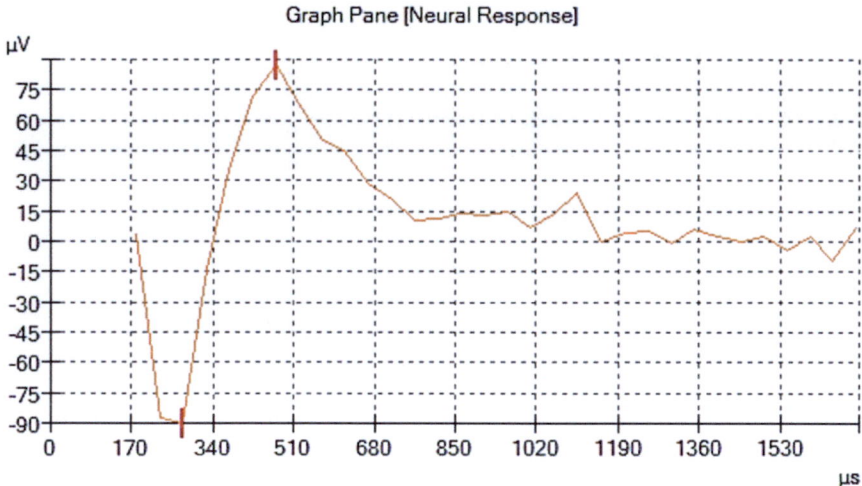

Fig. 5.10 Nerve action potential at the level of the middle cochlear turn; a proper depolarization of the nerve fibers can be confirmed

Case 5.2 *Right sided otosclerosis with ossification: subtotal petrosectomy with scala vestibuli insertion*

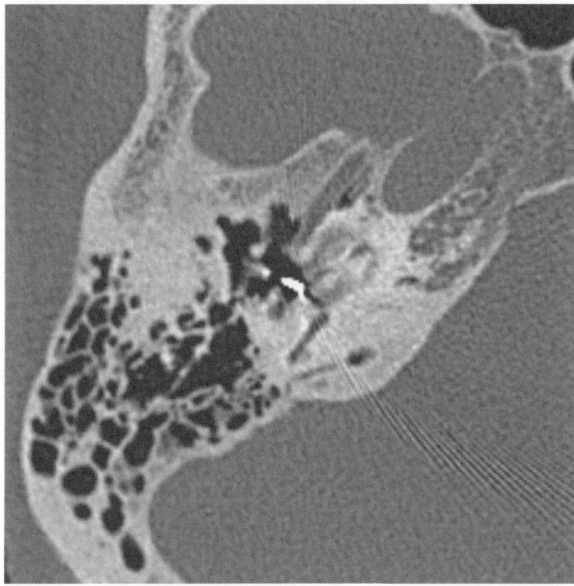

Fig. 5.11 Axial CT showing a significant otosclerotic rearrangement of the otic capsule. Note also the piston positioned in the previous surgery

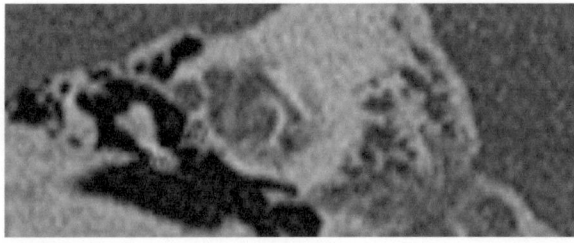

Fig. 5.12 The coronal section confirms the massive cochlear involvement

Fig. 5.13 Even with the improved view provided by the SP, both the RW and the OW cannot be clearly identified

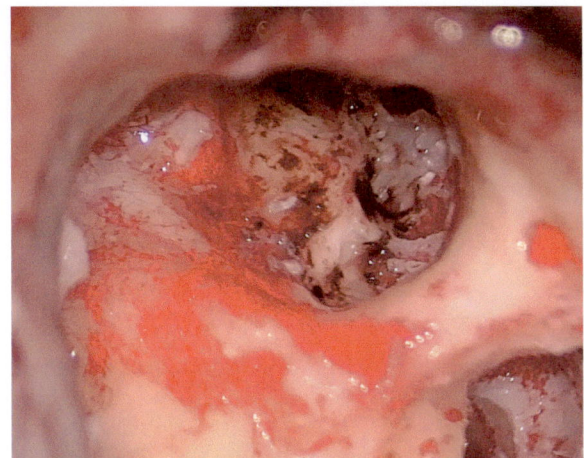

Fig. 5.14 Initial promontory drilling (black asterisk) is not able to provide access to the cochlear lumen

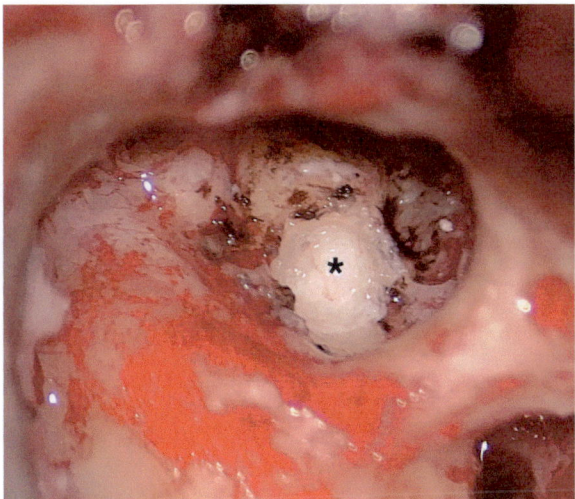

Fig. 5.15 Moving the drilling a bit superiorly allows identification of a dark area, probed with a hook

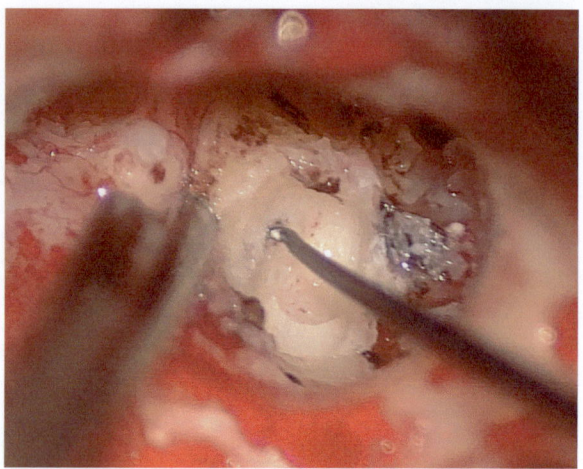

Fig. 5.16 The previous maneuver opens the cochlear lumen at the level of the scala vestibuli (white arrow)

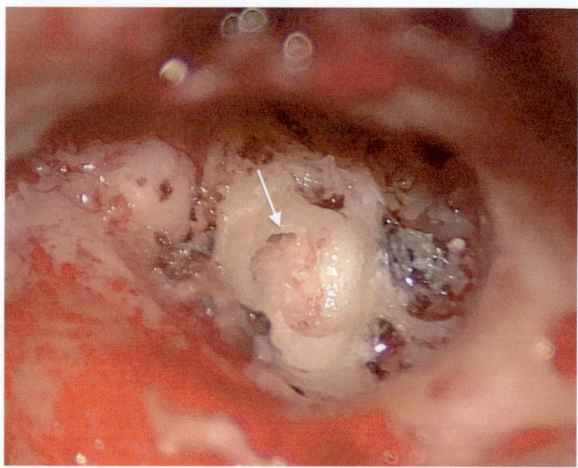

Fig. 5.17 The small opening is enlarged by means of a small diamond bur

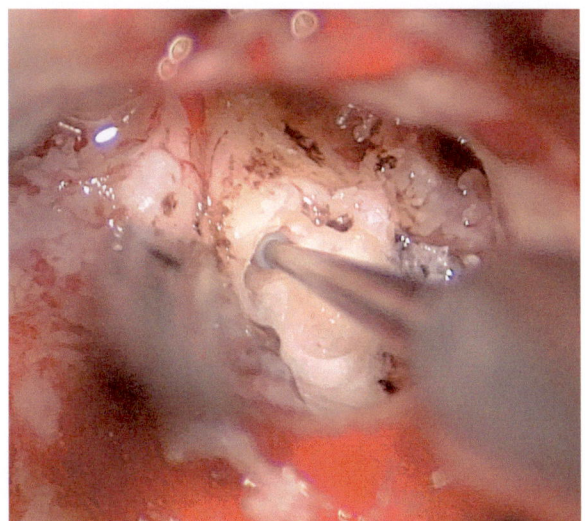

Fig. 5.18 Finally, the scala vestibuli is opened enough to accommodate the array. Note how far anterior the scala tympani was completely occluded (black asterisk)

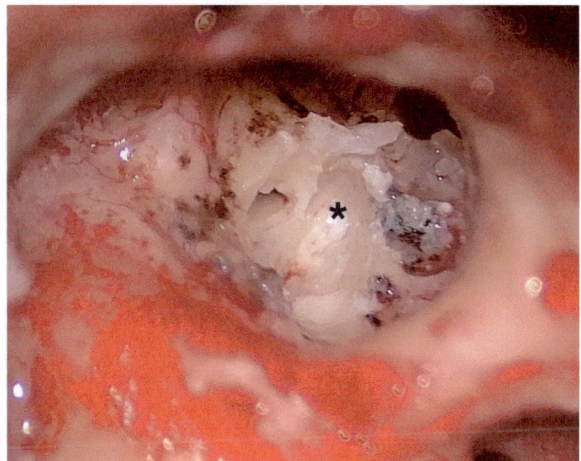

Fig. 5.19 The array is fully inserted into the scala vestibuli

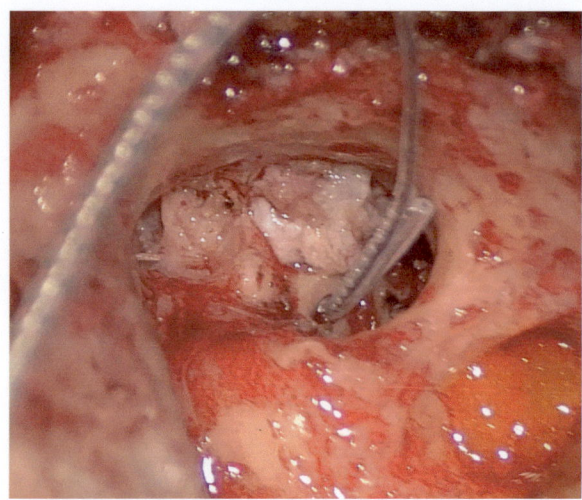

Fig. 5.20 Postoperative CT confirms the correct positioning of the array

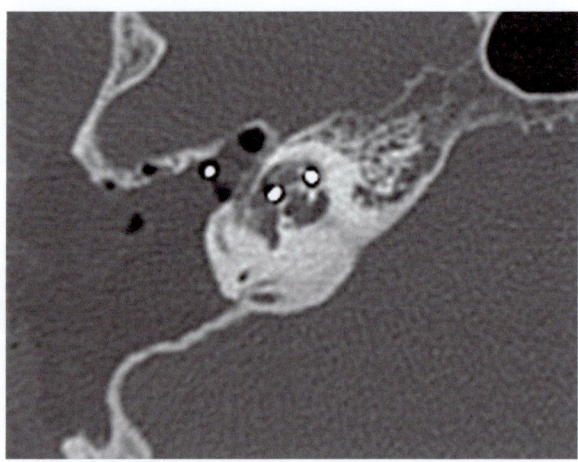

5 Cochlear Implantation in Advanced Otosclerosis

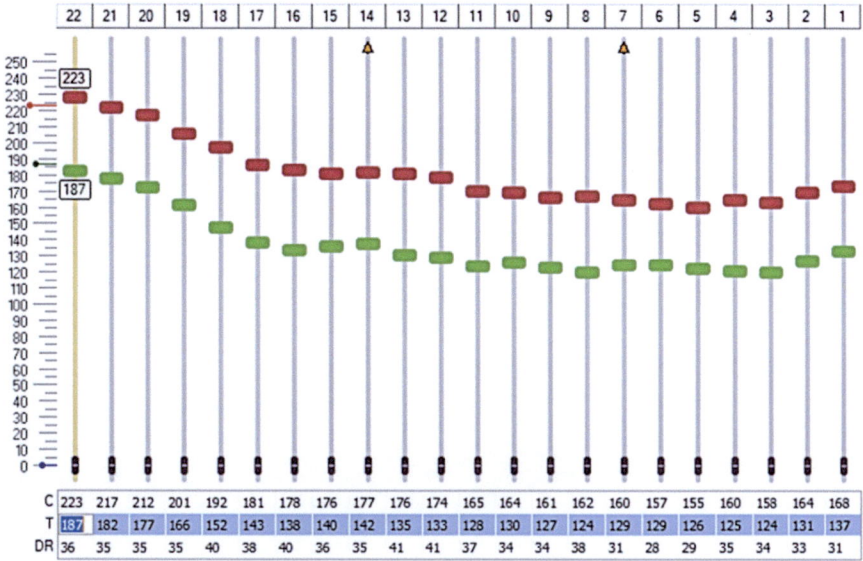

Fig. 5.21 Starting from electrode no. 18, a remarkable increase in stimulation levels can be seen, probably due to a scalar migration

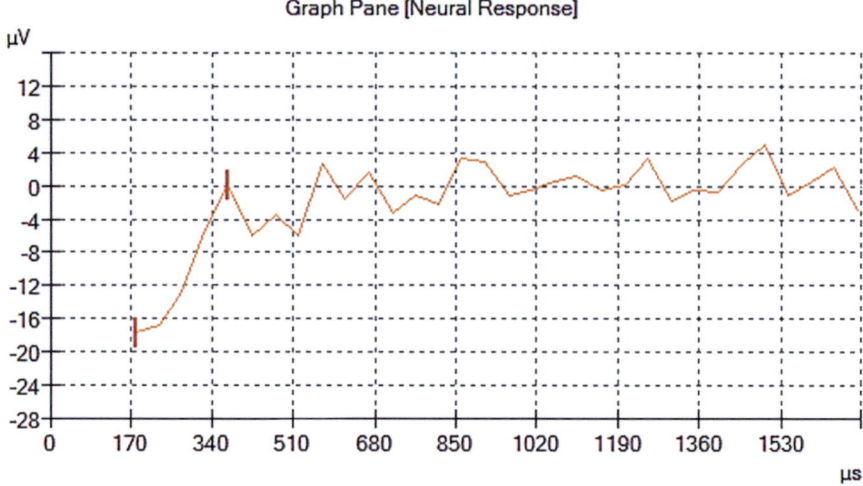

Fig. 5.22 At the level of the apical electrodes, it is not possible to record any clear nerve action potential because of the insertion trauma (electrode no. 20)

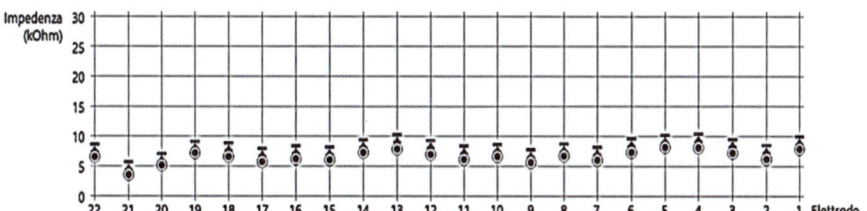

Fig. 5.23 No impedance modification can be seen even in the critical stimulation area

Case 5.3 *Left sided cavitary otosclerosis: subtotal petrosectomy with scala tympani insertion*

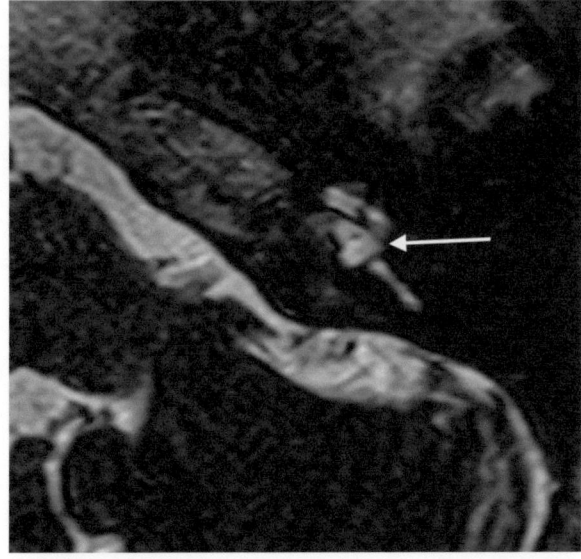

Fig. 5.24 MR showing an otosclerosis cavity (white arrow) involving the RW area

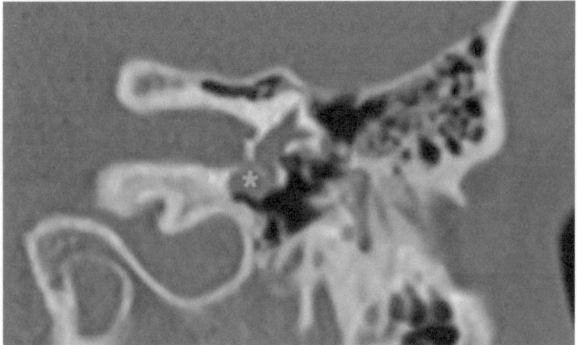

Fig. 5.25 The coronal CT confirms the cavitation (green asterisk) identified in the MR images

Fig. 5.26 Surgical approach through the SP. The presence of a hypotympanic cell may also be misleading

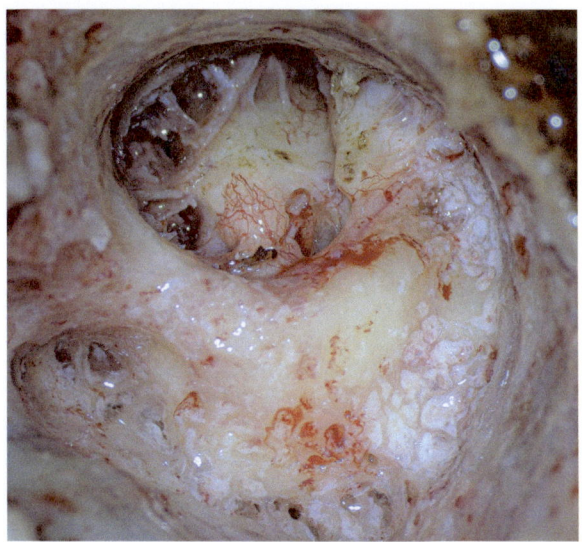

Fig. 5.27 Initial drilling in the supposed RW area allows to identify a large bluish area (black asterisk) inferiorly to the stapes

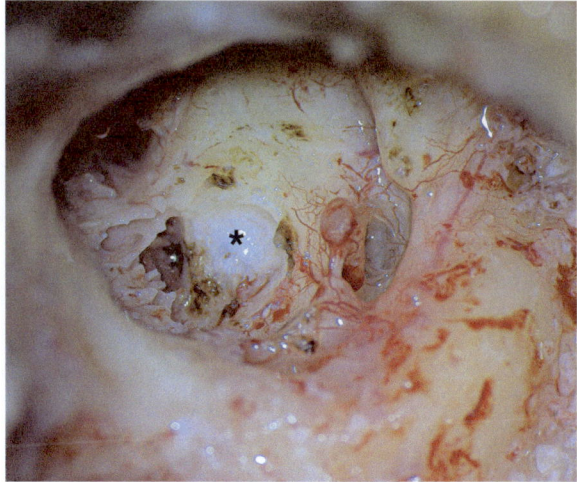

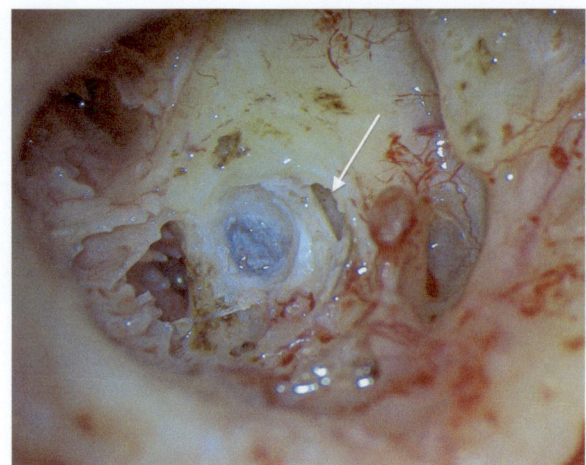

Fig. 5.28 The bluish area is better defined (cavitary otosclerosis?) and a smaller opening (white arrow) close to the stapes is also identified (scala vestibuli?)

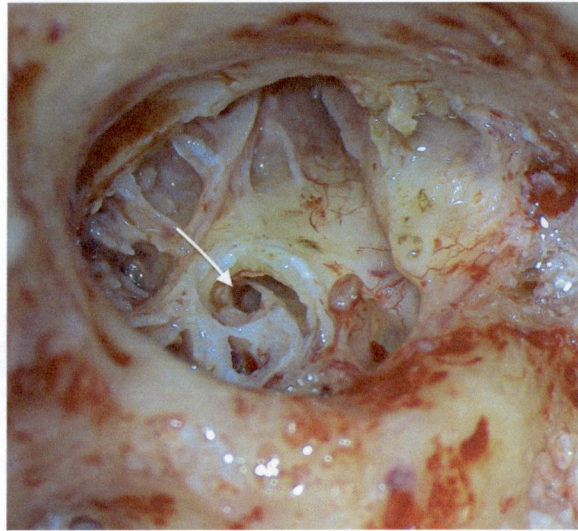

Fig. 5.29 Further drilling allows to clearly differentiate the otosclerosis cavitation from the cochlear lumen. The scala tympani (white arrow) has been calibrated to accommodate the array

5 Cochlear Implantation in Advanced Otosclerosis

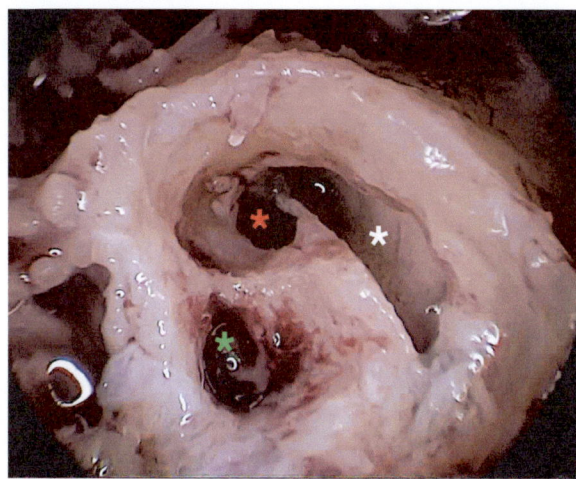

Fig. 5.30 Before array insertion, the beautiful inner anatomy of the cochlea is visualized with the help of an endoscope. The large otosclerosis cavity (green asterisk) postero-inferior to the scala tympani (red asterisk) could be easily interpreted as the scala tympani itself if working through the narrow and dark space offered by the posterior tympanotomy. The scala vestibuly is marked with a white asterisk

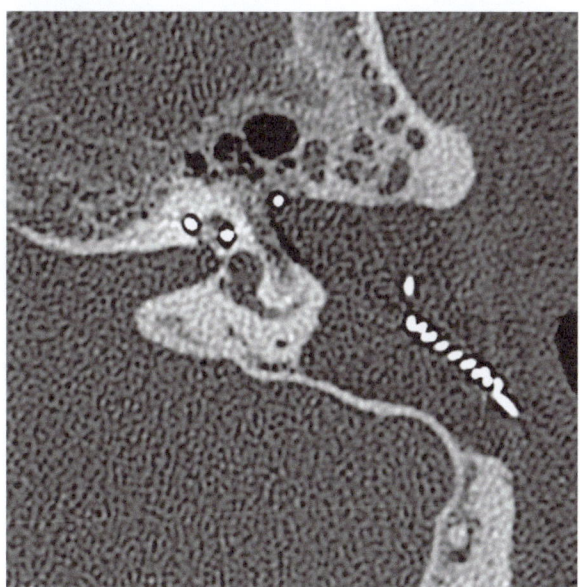

Fig. 5.31 Postop CT showing the array running correctly into the cochlear lumen

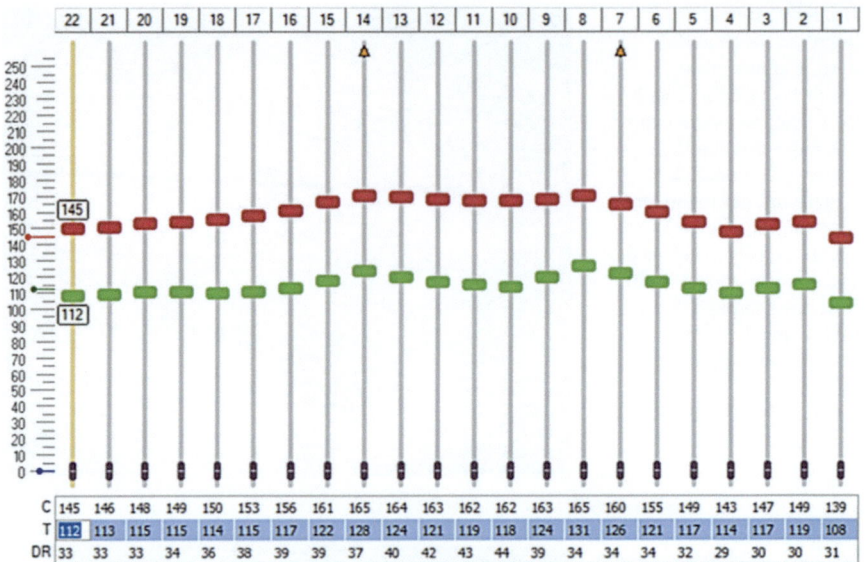

Fig. 5.32 Despite the drilling procedure, adequate levels of stimulation may be applied

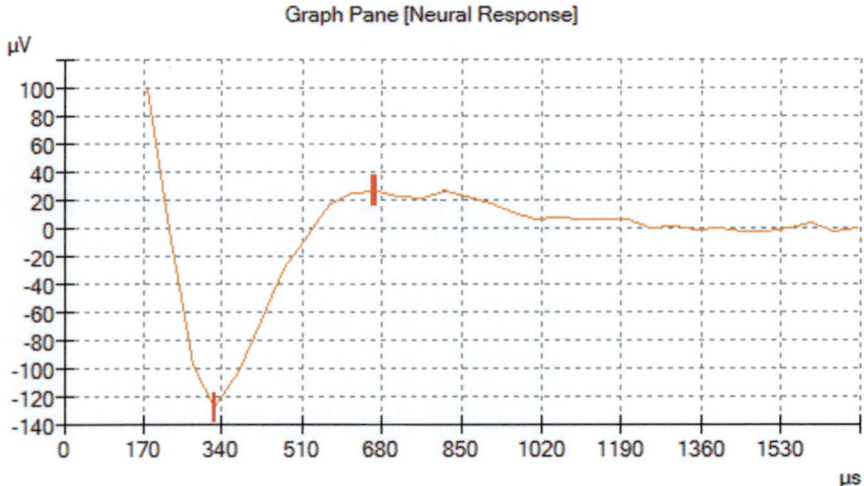

Fig. 5.33 The neural response is adequate too

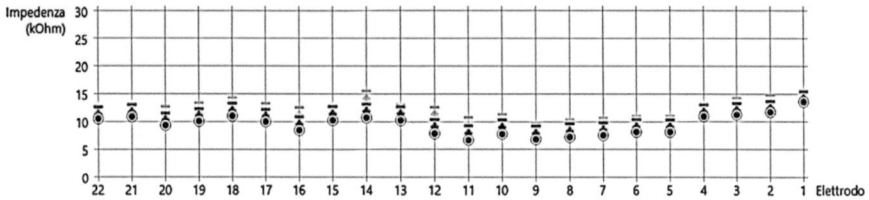

Fig. 5.34 Recorded impedances follow a linear pathway, within a normal range

References

1. Castillo F, et al. Cochlear implantation outcomes in advanced otosclerosis. Am J Otolaryngol. 2014;35(5):558–64. https://doi.org/10.1016/j.amjoto.2014.03.011.
2. Dumas AR, et al. Cochlear implantation in far-advanced otosclerosis: hearing results and complications. Acta Otorhinolaryngol Italica. 2018;38(5):445–52. https://doi.org/10.14639/0392-100x-1442.
3. Makarem AO, et al. Cavitating otosclerosis. Otology Neurotol. 2010;31(3):381–4. https://doi.org/10.1097/mao.0b013e3181d275e8.
4. Rotteveel LJ, et al. Cochlear implantation in 53 patients with otosclerosis: demographics, computed tomographic scanning, surgery, and complications. Otology Neurotol. 2004;25(6):943–52. https://doi.org/10.1097/00129492-200411000-00014.
5. Sanna M. Surgery for cochlear and other auditory implants, 2015. Stuttgart: Thieme; 2015.
6. D'Angelo G, et al. Subtotal petrosectomy and cochlear implantation. Acta Otorhinolaryngol Italica. 2020;40(6):450–6. https://doi.org/10.14639/0392-100x-n0931.
7. Issing PR, et al. Cochlear implantation in patients with chronic otitis: Indications for subtotal petrosectomy and obliteration of the Middle Ear. Skull Base. 1998;8(03):127–31. https://doi.org/10.1055/s-2008-1058571.
8. Free RH, et al. The role of subtotal petrosectomy in cochlear implant surgery–a report of 32 cases and review on indications. Otol Neurotol. 2013;34(6):1033–40. https://doi.org/10.1097/mao.0b013e318289841b.

Cochlear Implantation in Post-meningitis and Post-labyrinthitis Deafness

6

The main problem related to cochlear implantation (CI) in a deaf ear due to labyrinthitis and/or meningitis is related to the possible presence of cochlear fibrosis or, even worse, cochlear ossification [1, 2]. This latter may develop extremely fast so, as a general rule, these patients need to be implanted as soon as possible [3]. The amount of bony tissue in an ossified cochlea may not be sufficient to be clearly detected by the computed tomography (CT) scan [4], so this latter may underestimate the real involvement of the cochlea. As a consequence, whenever possible, the patient should undergo a preoperative magnetic resonance imaging (MRI) to better evaluate the presence and extension of the cochlear lumen available for implantation [5]. Differently from the otosclerosis, where the pattern of ossification is more regular, the position and extension of ossification after a labyrinthitis/meningitis are much less predictable. The majority of the cases the process starts in the basal turn and the scala tympani; however it is not uncommon to find patients with ossification extended to even to the scala vestibuli (Figs. 6.2, 6.3, 6.4, 6.5, and 6.6) as well as to the middle and apical turns (Figs. 6.17, 6.18, 6.19, 6.20, 6.21, 6.22, 6.23, 6.24, 6.25, and 6.26) [6]. Ossification confined to the upper portions of the cochlea is rarer but may also be present (Figs. 6.10, 6.11, 6.12, 6.13, and 6.14).

Two main criteria dictate the indication and approach in severely ossified ears: extent of the ossification and hearing status in the contralateral ear. A complete ossification ("white cochlea") (Fig. 6.1) is usually a contraindication to CI surgery. However, when the other ear is even in a similar situation, a CI attempt may be justified, before proceeding directly with an ABI [7].

As for the otosclerosis case, the use of short and rigid arrays, inserted with the stylet still in place, should be preferred. In severe ossification, the stylet may also be left into the cochlea, in order to facilitate the array extraction if an explanation is required in the future. Furthermore, the use of a depth gauge as a dummy array is advised before the real insertion. Even in this situation, as well as in the otosclerosis cases, the scala vestibuli insertion can be considered as a possible option in those

Fig. 6.1 CT, showing a complete ossification (red arrow), commonly defined "white cochlea"

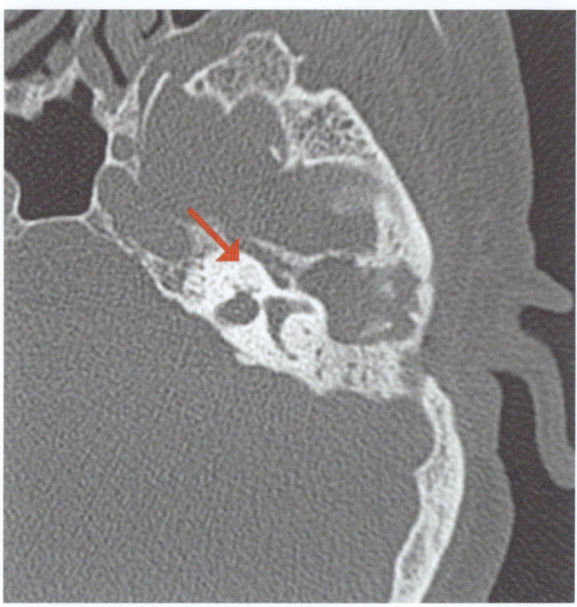

cases in which after a proper drill-out of the scala timpani, no visible cochlear lumen could be detected [8].

In all these postoperative cases, CT scan is mandatory to confirm the correct array insertion (Figs. 6.7, 6.14, and 6.26).

Hearing rehabilitation results following cochlear implantation in patients with post-meningitis/-labyrinthitis cochlear ossification are heterogeneous. In addition to the aggressive surgery required, the ossification itself may produce different patterns of destruction of the neural ganglion cells. Those factors should be preoperatively evaluated through a proper electrophysiological testing, such as to communicate to the patient the hypothetical expectations derived from the cochlear implantation procedure.

As for the otosclerosis cases, postoperative mapping (Figs. 6.8, 6.9, 6.15, 6.16, 6.26, 6.27, and 6.28) may present additional difficulties; even in some of these patients, it can be helpful to rely on a different intracochlear stimulation modalities (pseudo-monopolar, bipolar, bipolar +1...) in order to reduce the electrical stimulation diffusion and the related facial nerve stimulation.

Case 6.1 Post-meningitis basal turn ossification.

Fig. 6.2 CT, showing an apparently mild ossification limited to the beginning of the basal turn (red arrow). The patient could not undergo an MRI, because of the presence of an old implant (not MRI compatible) on the other side

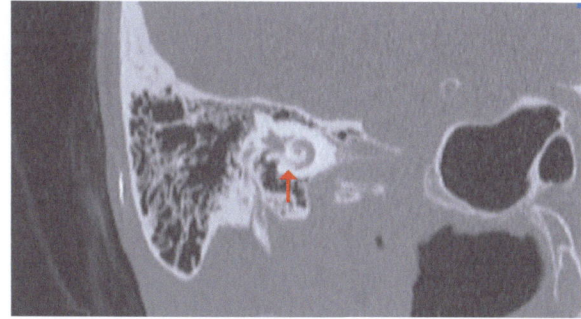

Fig. 6.3 View of the surgical field after SP and initial drill-out (black asterisk)

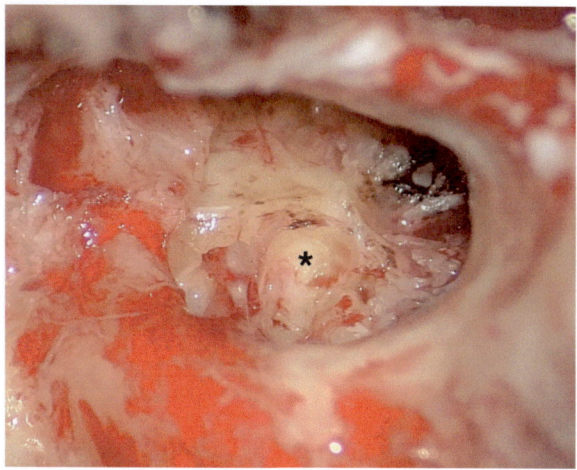

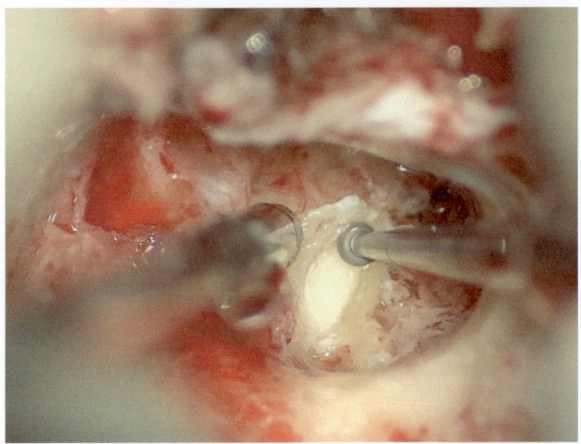

Fig. 6.4 Further drilling clearly allows to identify the whitish post-meningitis ossification

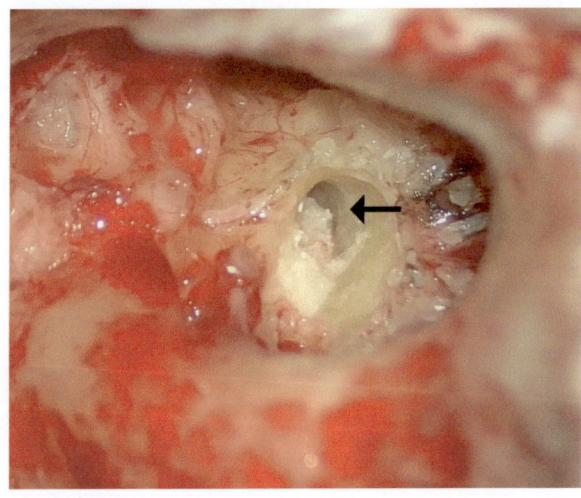

Fig. 6.5 After drilling, the majority of the inferior half of the basal turn of a cochlear lumen is identified and a large cochleostomy accomplished (black arrow), encompassing both the scala tympani and vestibuli

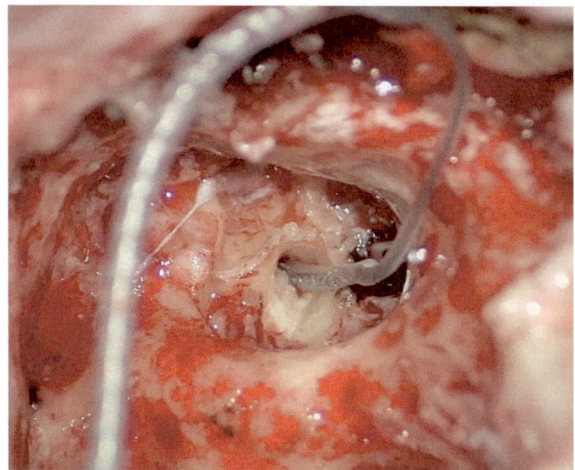

Fig. 6.6 After checking the cochlear lumen with a depth gauge, the real array is fully inserted

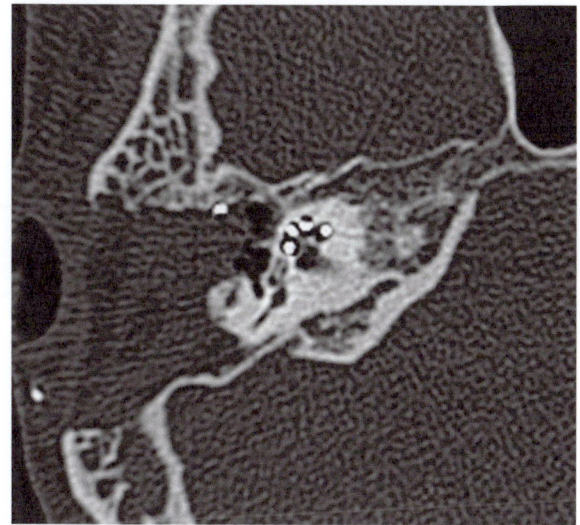

Fig. 6.7 Postop CT scan, showing the intracochlear position of the array. Because of the position of the cochleostomy at the far end of the anterior half of the basal turn, the tip of the array (even if a short one) reaches the apical turn

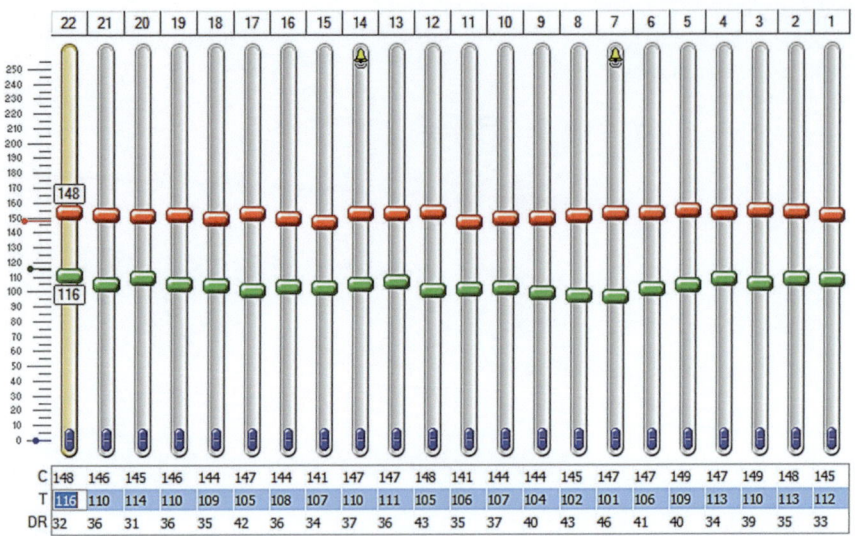

Fig. 6.8 After bypassing the critical area, the remaining cochlea seems be able to be stimulated in standard situation

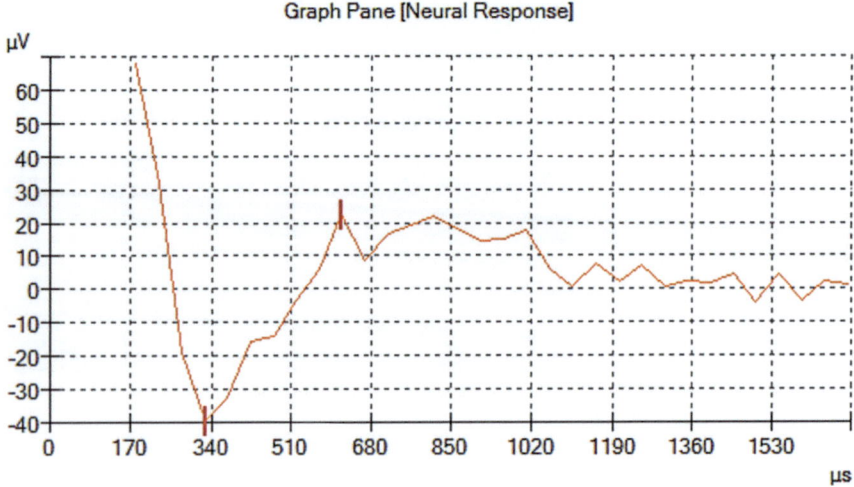

Fig. 6.9 A sufficient depolarizations is obtained even if with a reduced amplitude of the neural response. This can also be influenced by the long deprivation (about 30 years)

Case 6.2 Post-meningitis middle and apical turn ossification.

Fig. 6.10 MR showing absence of fluid in the middle and apical turn of the cochlea

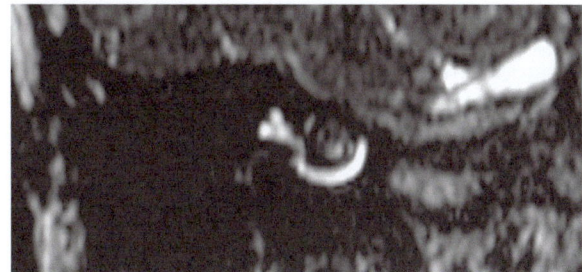

Fig. 6.11 Reconstructed CT confirming that the basal turn seems available for implantation, while the most apical area of the cochlear lumen is ossified (red arrow)

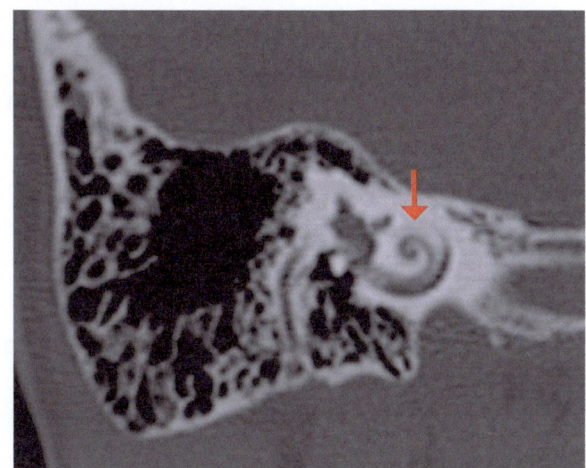

Fig. 6.12 After the SP has been completed, unexpected ossification is found in the RW area (black asterisk)

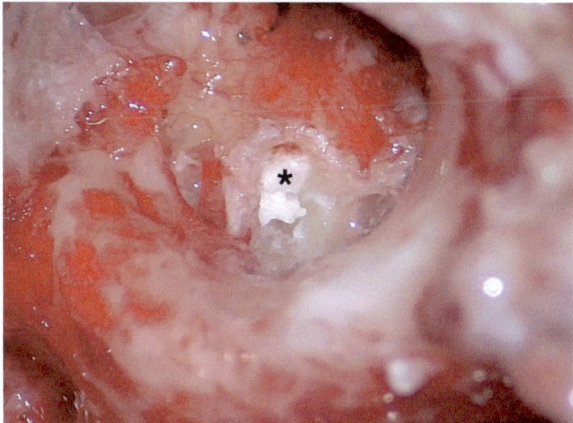

Fig. 6.13 After complete exposure of the cochlear lumen, insertion of a depth gauge confirms the possibility to insert 18 electrodes into the cochlea

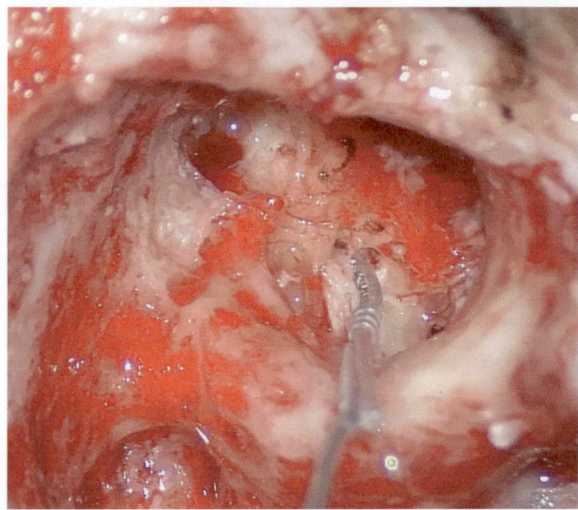

Fig. 6.14 Postop CT showing the partial insertion

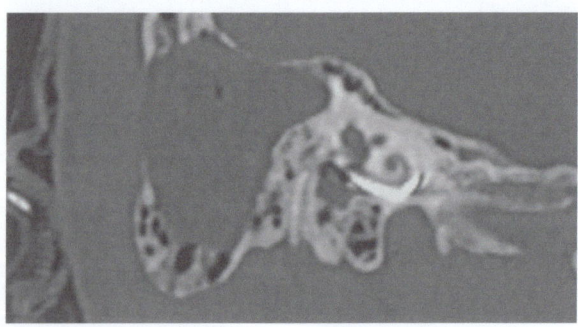

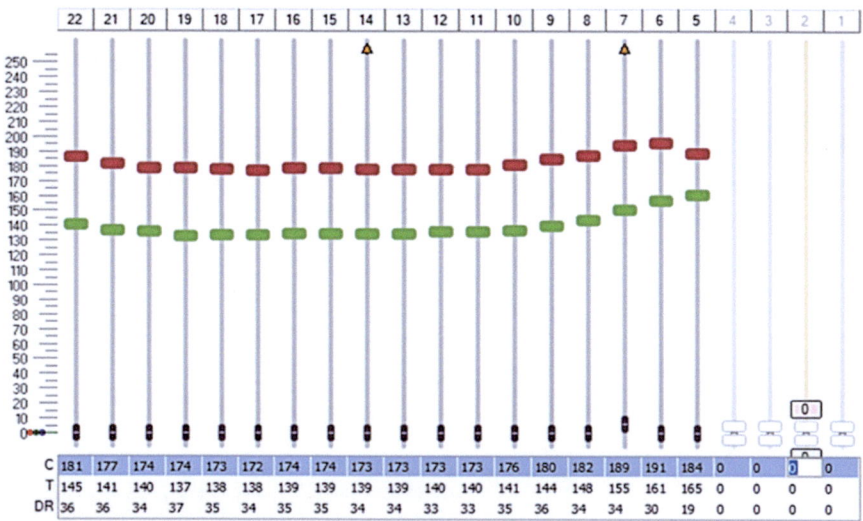

Fig. 6.15 As a consequence of the incomplete insertions, the map of the stimulation levels is limited to 18 electrodes

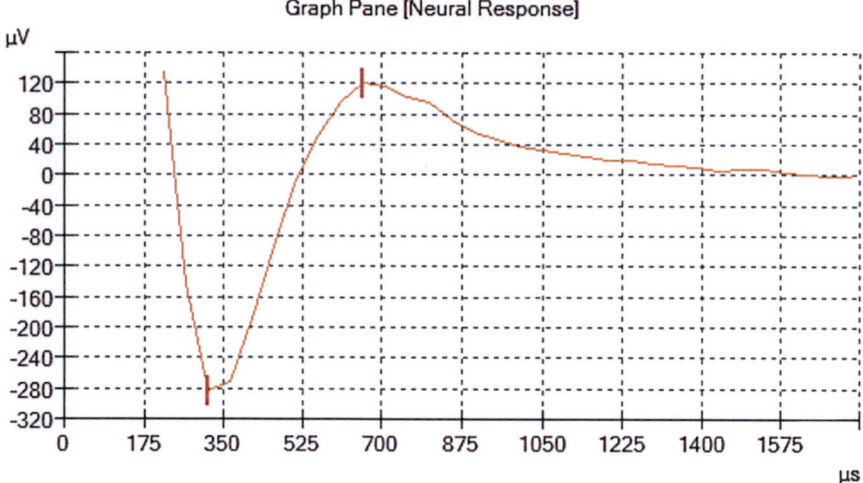

Fig. 6.16 The nerve action potential shows good morphology, amplitude, and latency for all the active electrodes, a crucial factor to obtain good functional results

Case 6.3 Post-meningitis subtotal ossification, contralateral CI not MRI compatible with initial soft failure.

Fig. 6.17 CT reconstruction showing the entire cochlear shape and the extent of ossification

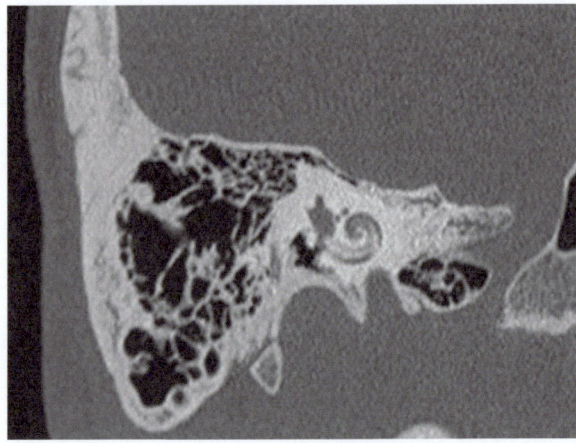

Fig. 6.18 After drilling of the basal turn, exposure of the cochlear (white arrow) seems achieved

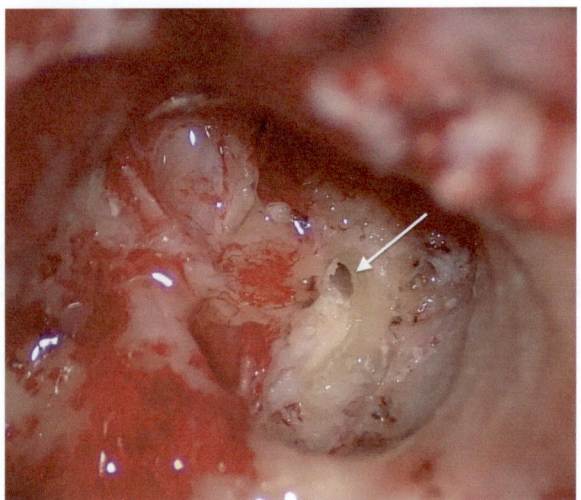

Fig. 6.19 An attempt to insert a depth gauge encounters an obstacle after only a few electrodes

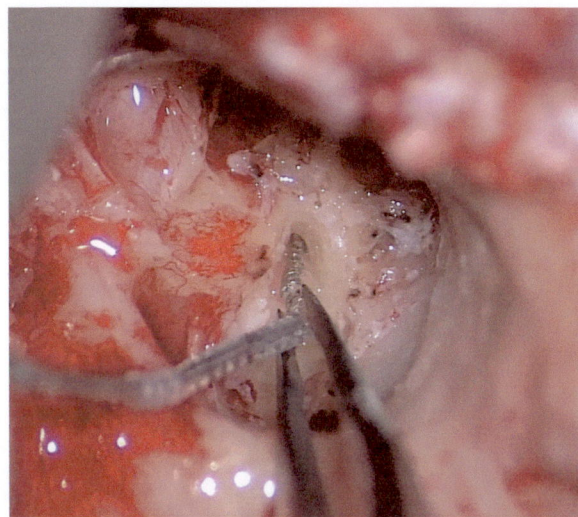

Fig. 6.20 Addition drilling of the basal turn does not offer any advantage

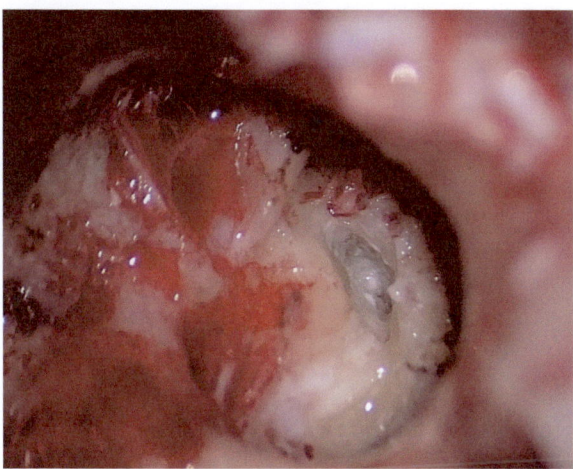

Fig. 6.21 A decision is taken to try to identify the middle turn, drilling the promontorium anterior to the stapes

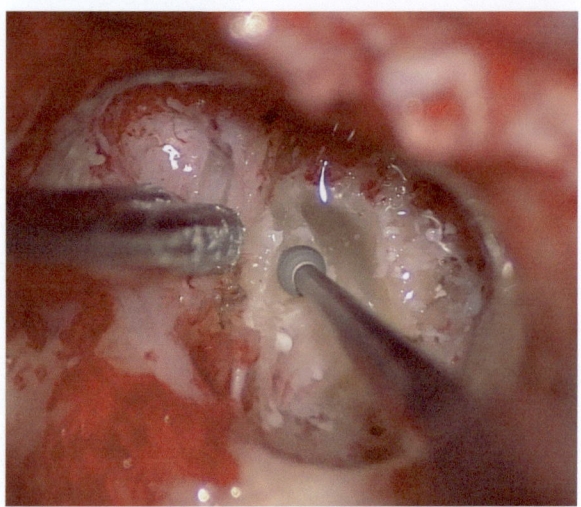

Fig. 6.22 The middle turn (white arrow) is opened in its most superior extension

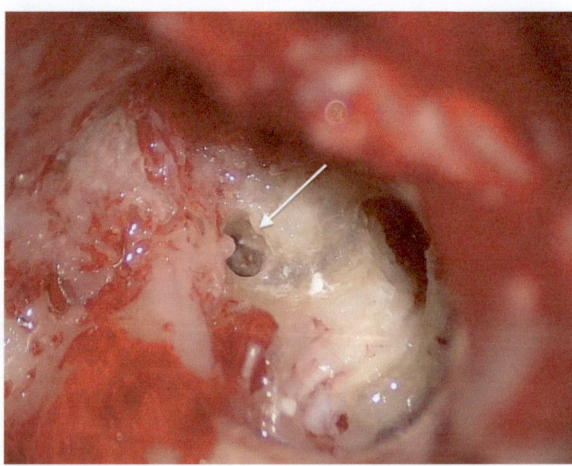

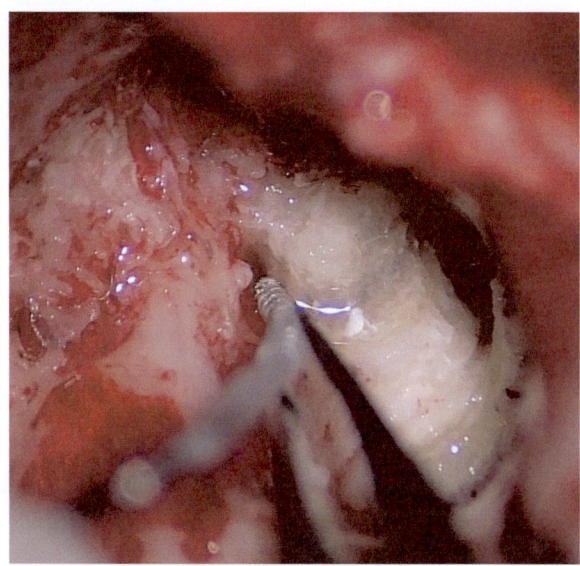

Fig. 6.23 Another attempt to get in position enough electrodes of a depth gauge, this time in a retrograde fashion starting from the middle turn, fails again

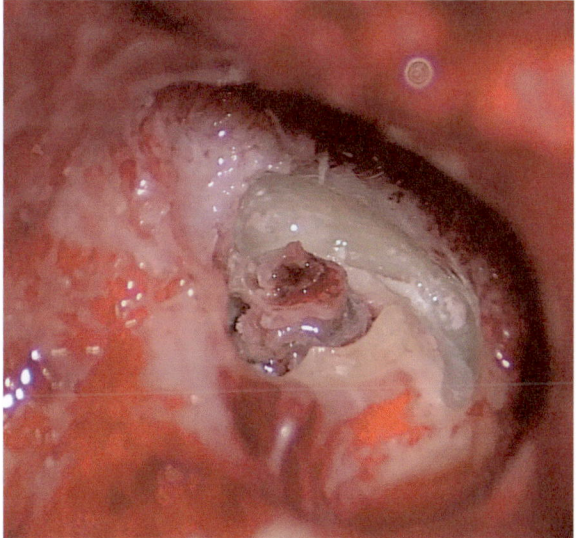

Fig. 6.24 A total drill-out is finally performed, exposing all the cochlear turns

Fig. 6.25 The real array is positioned in the groove drilled all around the modiolus

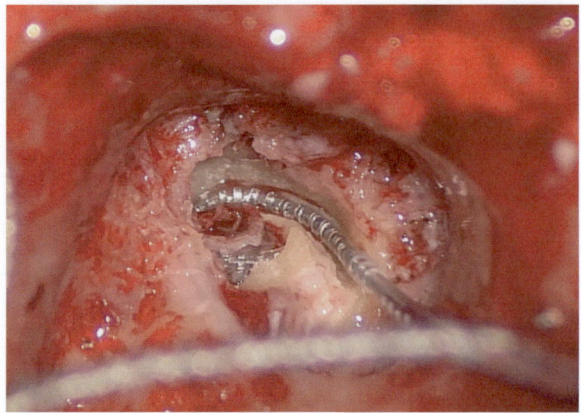

Fig. 6.26 Reconstruction of the CT along the cochlea plane allows to better estimate the position of the array. Note the vicinity of the drilling to the carotid canal (white asterisk)

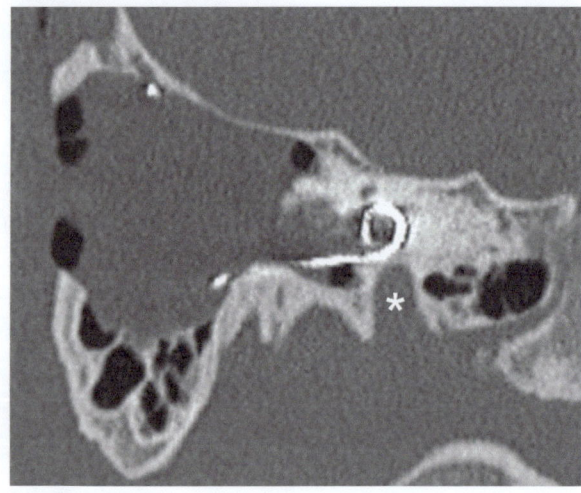

6 Cochlear Implantation in Post-meningitis and Post-labyrinthitis Deafness

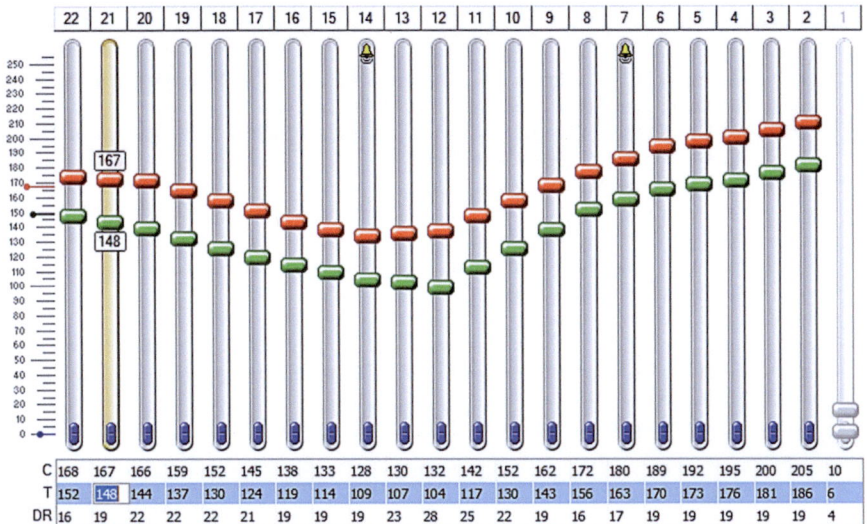

Fig. 6.27 By adopting a pseudomonopolar intracochlear stimulation modality, it was possible to activate all the electrodes. In spite of the high stimulation levels required to obtain a hearing sensation, no facial nerve activation was elicited

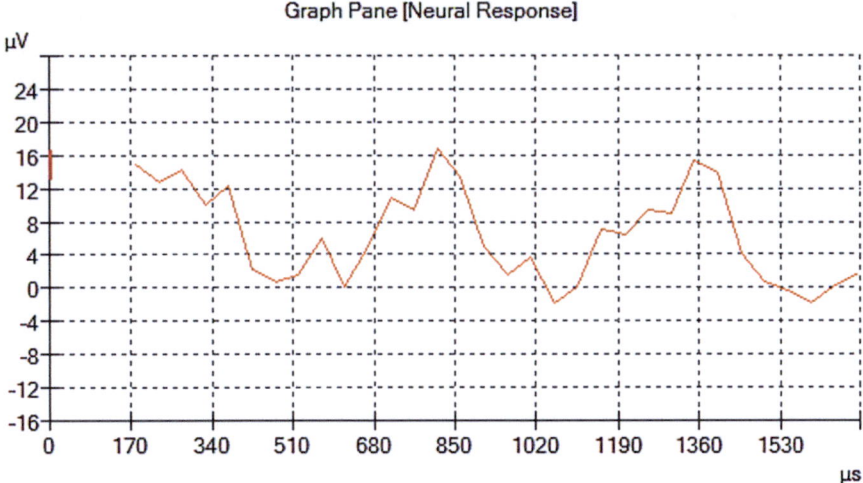

Fig. 6.28 Notwithstanding the high levels of stimulation, the nerve action potential was not elicited by any electrode. This was probably the consequence of the obstacle represented by the amount of residual bone for the electrical stimuli to reach the residual ganglia fibers. The absence of sufficient neural depolarization did not allow the patient to reach an open-set recognition, but only some words identification

References

1. Alanazi GA, Alrashidi AS, Alqarni KS, Khozym SAA, Alenzi S. Meningitis post-cochlear implant and role of vaccination. Saudi Med J. 2022;43(12):1300–8.
2. O'Donoghue G, Balkany T, Cohen N, Lenarz T, Lustig L, Niparko J. Meningitis and cochlear implantation. Otol Neurotol. 2002;23(6):823–4.
3. Sanna M. Surgery for cochlear and other auditory implants, 2015. Stuttgart: Thieme; 2015.
4. Swartz JD, Loevner LA. Imaging of the temporal bone. New York: Thieme; 2009.
5. van Loon MC, et al. Magnetic resonance imaging in the evaluation of patients with sensorineural hearing loss caused by meningitis. Otol Neurotol. 2013;34(5):845–54. https://doi.org/10.1097/mao.0b013e31828dafee.
6. Schuknecht HF. Pathology of the ear. Philadelphia: Lea & Febiger; 1993.
7. Merkus P, et al. Indications and contraindications of auditory brainstem implants: systematic review and illustrative cases. Eur Arch Oto Rhino Laryngol. 2013;271(1):3–13. https://doi.org/10.1007/s00405-013-2378-3.
8. Pruitt P. Imaging of the temporal bone DeckerMed Otolaryngol 2020.

Simple Chronic Otitis and Cochlear Implantation

7

Application of the standard cochlear implant (CI) technique in the presence of a simple chronic otitis may require two surgical procedures (a miringoplasty followed by the cochlear implantation), with the subsequent risk of recurrence and the need for an additional revision surgery. If the SP is selected as surgical approach, the procedure may be performed in a single stage, even canceling the risk of perforation recurrence; for this reason, it is usually the approach adopted in this situation by the majority of the surgeons [1].

From a technical point of view, it is possible to distinguish among (1) chronic otitis with no or mild active infection and (2) chronic otitis with severe active infection.

In the first case, mainly a simple dry tympanic membrane perforation, the surgical steps follow exactly those described in Chap. 2 (the case in fact describes a simple tympanic perforation, see Figs. 2.3, 2.4, 2.5, 2.6, 2.7, 2.8, 2.9, 2.10, 2.11, 2.12, 2.13, 2.14, 2.15, 2.16, 2.17, 2.18, 2.19, 2.20, 2.21, 2.22, and 2.23).

In the presence of a severe active infection (e.g., osteoradionecrosis as in Figs. 7.1 and 7.2), particular care must be reserved to removing/cauterizing as much mucosa as possible, in order to minimize the risk of a postoperative cavity infection (Figs. 7.3 and 7.4) [2]. The possibility of performing a staged procedure must be taken into account intraoperatively, particularly in cases in which the surgeon does not feel confident with the extent and completeness of the disease removal [3]. If the staged option is selected, sometimes it can be indicated to avoid the obliteration of the cavity with fat during the first stage, due to its elevated risk of postoperative infection. The second stage is usually performed after at least 3 months [4].

From a technical point of view, when the obliteration of cavity using abdominal fat has been performed during the first stage, it is not necessary to completely remove it during the second stage, because there is no need to access again the anterior portion of the middle ear cleft [5]. Reopening of the mastoid (Figs. 7.5 and 7.6) and visualization of the RW area (Fig. 7.7) are usually sufficient to safely insert the array (Fig. 7.8).

© The Author(s), under exclusive license to Springer Nature Switzerland AG 2025
M. Falcioni et al., *Cochlear Implant - Rare and Difficult Cases*, https://doi.org/10.1007/978-3-032-02323-0_7

Case 7.1 *Simple tympanic membrane perforation (see Chap. 2, Figs. 2.3, 2.4, 2.5, 2.6, 2.7, 2.8, 2.9, 2.10, 2.11, 2.12, 2.13, 2.14, 2.15, 2.16, 2.17, 2.18, 2.19, 2.20, 2.21, 2.22, and 2.23)*

Case 7.2 *Chronic otitis with severe active infection in radionecrosis (staged procedure)*

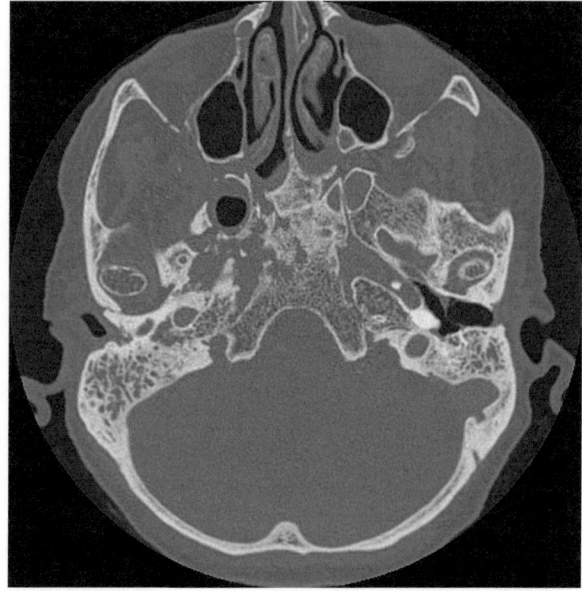

Fig. 7.1 Preoperative axial CT showing the severe necrosis of the clivus and the petrous bone after previous radiation therapy for nasopharyngeal carcinoma

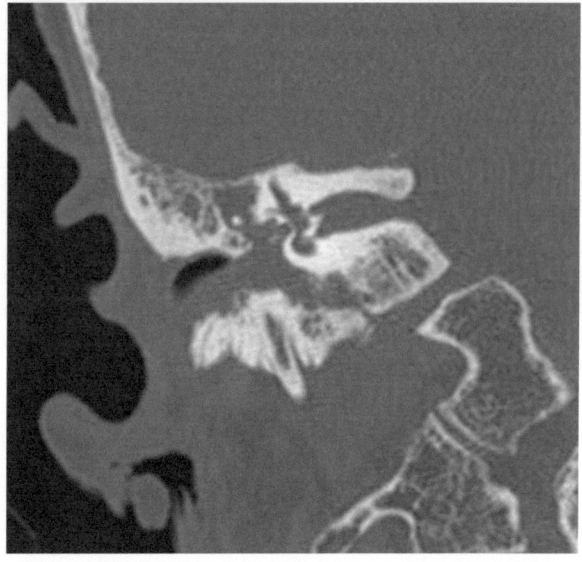

Fig. 7.2 Preoperative coronal CT showing involvement of the attic and the middle ear cleft, as well as necrosis of the inferior wall of the tympanic bone

Fig. 7.3 Stage 1; during the bony drilling, infected tissue is found in all the middle ear cleft and the mastoid

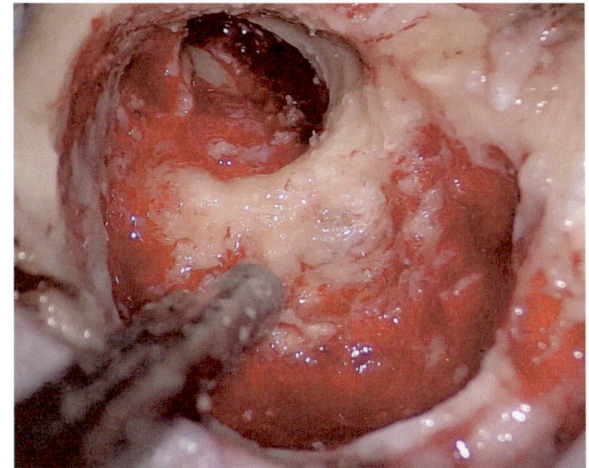

Fig. 7.4 Stage 1; aspect of the surgical cavity after bony work and disease removal. The inflammatory tissue has been completely removed/coagulated. The Eustachian tube has already been packed with muscle (black asterisk). However, due to the aggressiveness of the specific disease in this case, it was considered safer to stage the positioning of the implant

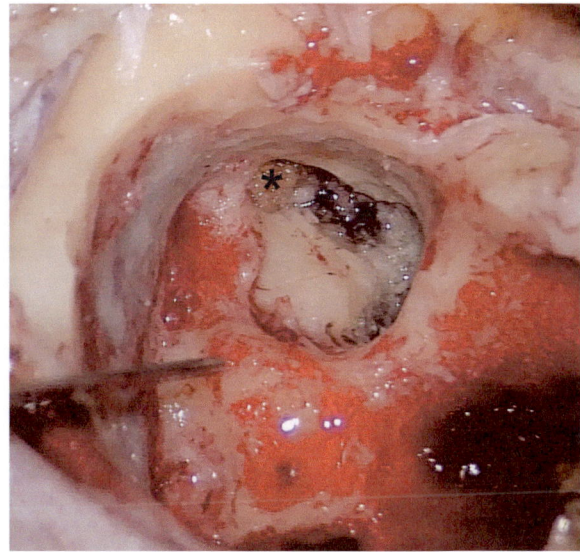

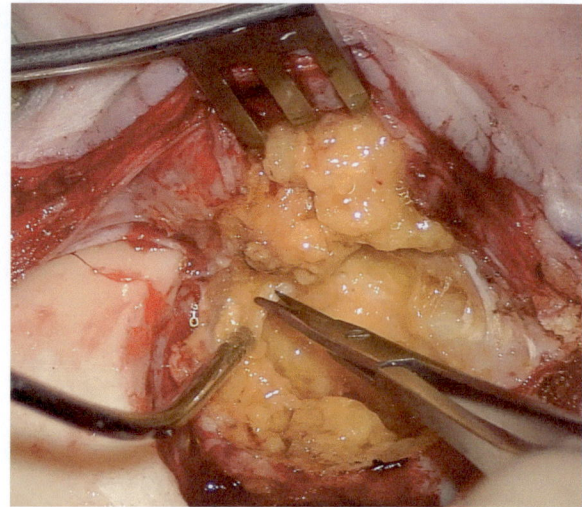

Fig. 7.5 Stage 2; after reopening of the previous wound, the fat filling the posterior aspect of the cavity is sectioned and progressively removed in order to locate the bony landmarks of the surgical cavity

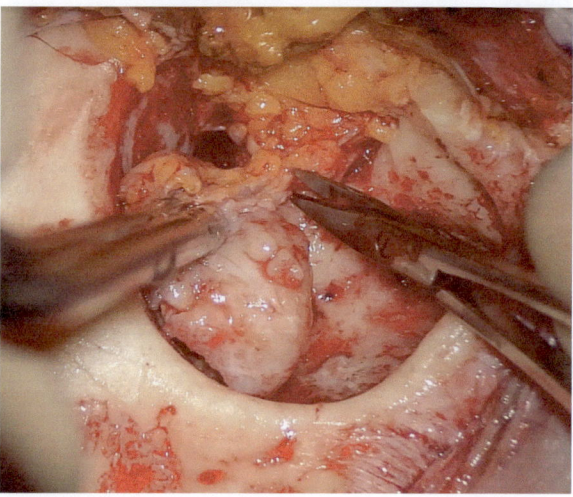

Fig. 7.6 Stage 2; removal of the fat filling the posterior aspect of the cavity allows identification of the postero-medial bony surface

7 Simple Chronic Otitis and Cochlear Implantation

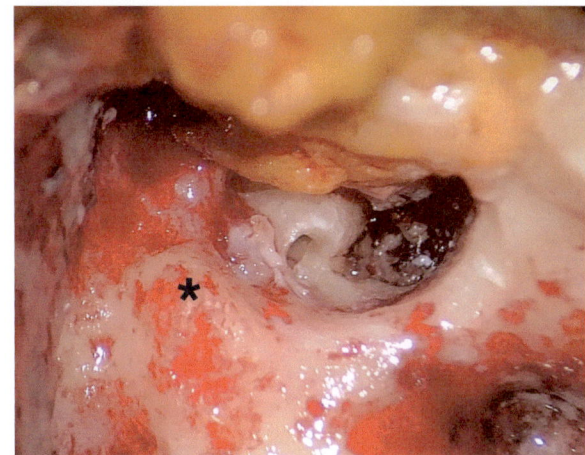

Fig. 7.7 Stage 2; after visualization of the lateral semicircular canal (black asterisk), the middle ear cleft is entered and the RW identified and opened. The anterior portion of the fat is left in place and the Eustachian tube orifice (already plugged) left undisturbed

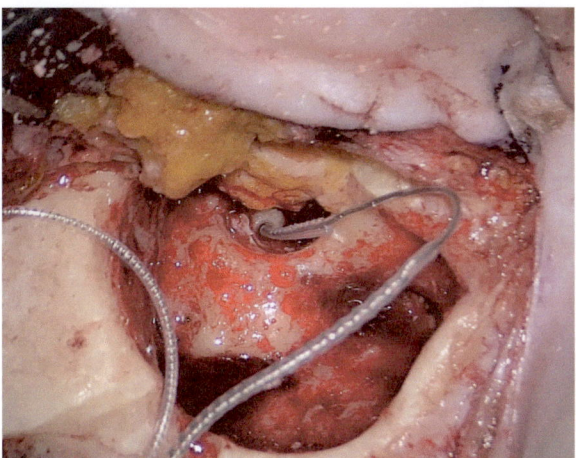

Fig. 7.8 Stage 2; a full array insertion is achieved. The posterior aspect of the cavity is then re-obliterated with fresh abdominal fat

References

1. Szymański M, Ataide A, Linder T. The use of subtotal petrosectomy in cochlear implant candidates with chronic otitis media. Eur Arch Otorhinolaryngol. 2016;273, fasc. 2:363–70. https://doi.org/10.1007/s00405-015-3573-1.
2. Shelton C, Sheehy JL. Tympanoplasty. Laryngoscope. 1990;100(7):679–81.
3. Sanna M. Middle ear and mastoid microsurgery. Thieme; 2003.
4. Sanna M, Sunose H, Mancini F, Russo A, Taibah A. Microsurgical management of middle ear and petrous bone cholesteatoma. Thieme; 2019.
5. Sadé J, Berco E, Buyanover D, Brown ML. Ossicular damage in chronic middle ear inflammation. Acta Otolaryngol. 1981;92(1–6):273–83.

Cochlear Implant Surgery in the Context of Cholesteatoma

8

Cholesteatoma is a chronic disease capable of recurrence even after many decades. This means that application of the standard cochlear implantation (CI) technique in cases of chronic otitis media with cholesteatoma results in a high percentage of recurrence of the pathology and subsequent malfunctioning of the device, with the need for revision surgery [1].

The general agreement advices to rely on the subtotal petrosectomy (SP) approach in those cases [2], even if with a few specific adaptations. Cholesteatoma removal must be performed carefully in order to reduce the chance of residual lesion. Whenever possible, the matrix should be dissected away without fragmentation and the bony areas in contact with the matrix drilled aggressively to reduce the risk of any remnants. If the cholesteatoma is in contact with soft tissue (i.e., the dura), this latter is better cauterized with the bipolar to have an additional safety concerning a complete disease removal [3].

Many other factors may be advocated as to underline the importance of SP in cholesteatoma cases, in addition to just the risk of leaving some matrix debris into the surgical cavity. Opening the cochlear lumen in the presence of an infected ear, in fact, increases the risk of a labyrinthitis and, as a consequence, of a potential intradural contamination. Furthermore, the profound hearing loss in those patients is often not directly related to the cholesteatoma itself but to previous surgical procedures, hence additional difficulties related to the distorted anatomy and the presence of some sort of cochlear ossifications may be often encountered.

Different scenarios, all of them relatively rare, of patients affected by chronic cholestetomatous otitis and requiring a CI may be encountered; they include:

- CI in acquired middle ear cholesteatoma
- CI in recurrent middle ear cholesteatoma after a canal wall-up (Figs. 8.1, 8.2, 8.3, 8.4, 8.5, 8.6, and 8.7)

- CI in recurrent middle ear cholesteatoma after a canal wall-down (Figs. 8.8, 8.9, 8.10, 8.11, 8.12, and 8.13)
- CI in residual middle ear cholesteatoma after a canal wall-up (Figs. 8.14, 8.15, 8.16, 8.17, 8.18, and 8.19)

As already discussed in the previous chapter, even in presence of a cholesteatoma, the CI insertion may be performed in the same stage with the disease removal or postponed to a second stage, depending on the severity of infection, the risk of residual lesions, and the personal philosophy of the surgeon [4]. However, if the target of staging is the disclosure of a small residual lesions, the second stage should be performed not earlier than 10 months after the first surgery, which represents a long delay for patients waiting for a hearing rehabilitation [5, 6]. For this reason, the authors usually prefer a single-stage surgery (Figs. 8.7 and 8.13). However, the final decision can also be taken intraoperatively, when disease removal has been accomplished. Because of the potential need of a postoperative RMI during the follow-up, the receiver-stimulator must be positioned as far as possible from the surgical cavity in order to have the center of the artifact as far away as possible from the target area [7, 8]. In presence of a recurrent cholesteatoma after a canal wall-down with a large meatoplasty, the blindsac closure of the EAC will also require some adjustments, as described in the next chapter (see Chap. 10, CI in previous canal wall-down).

Case 8.1 Recurrent cholesteatoma after canal wall-up tympanoplasty

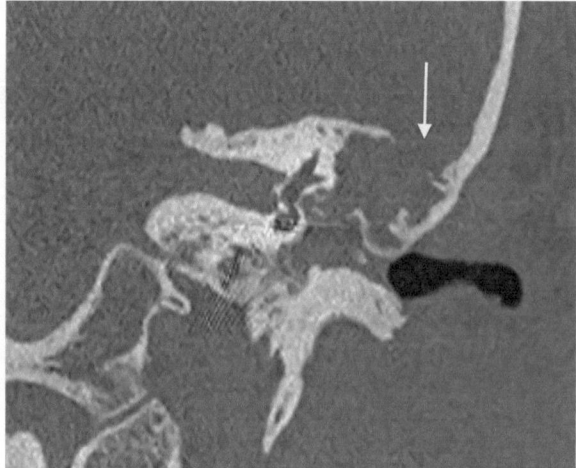

Fig. 8.1 Preoperative coronal CT showing a huge recurrent cholesteatoma with a large area of MCF dura exposed (white arrow)

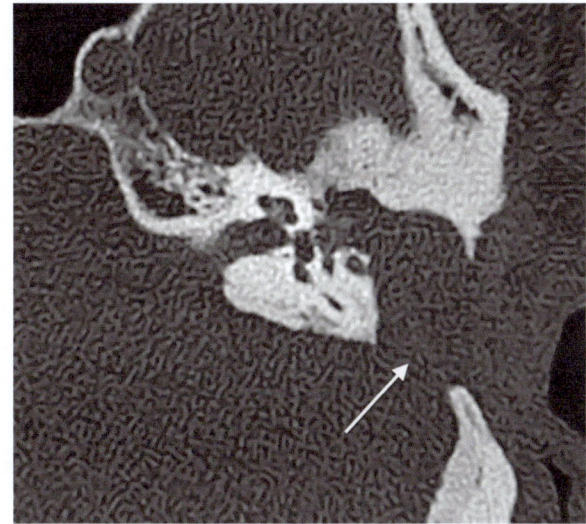

Fig. 8.2 Preoperative axial CT showing even an exposure of the sigmoid sinus (white arrows) and the posterior fossa dura. The inner ear appears intact, without any sign of ossification

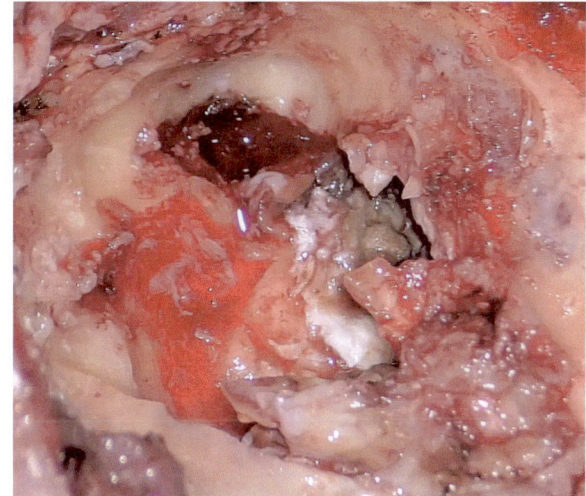

Fig. 8.3 At the beginning of the surgery, the previous mastoid cavity is found completely filled by scar/inflammatory tissue. Removal of this tissue and initial drilling of the posterior wall of the EAC allows visualization of the cholesteatoma involving the antrum and the attic

Fig. 8.4 In the middle ear cleft, the windows area is occupied by inflammatory tissue

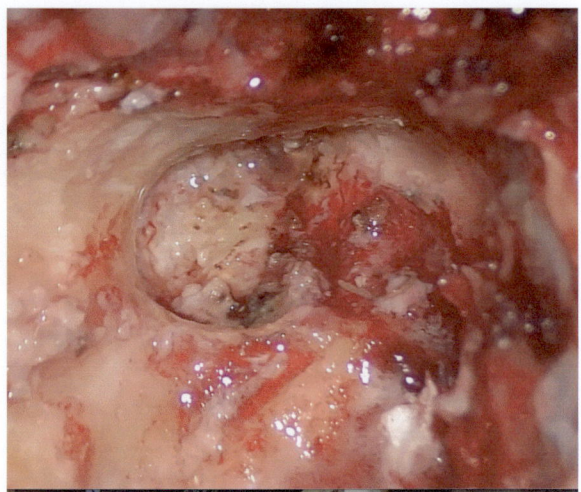

Fig. 8.5 After matrix removal, the exposed dura (white asterisk) has been gently coagulated in order to reduce the risk of skin remnants at this level

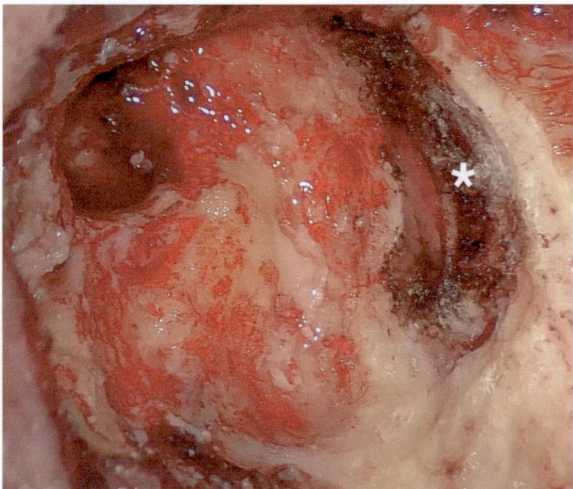

Fig. 8.6 Once the disease is completely removed, the round window (white arrow) is identified and opened

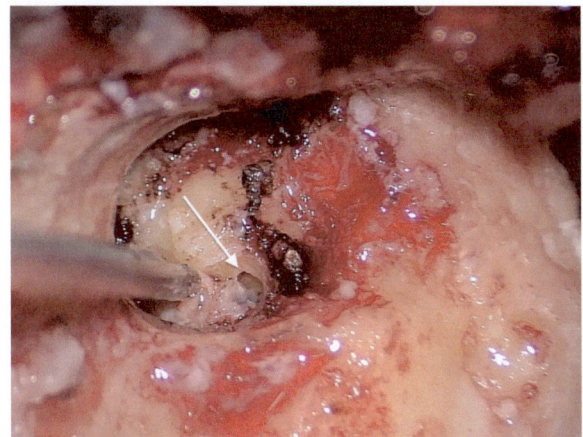

Fig. 8.7 The CI array is easily introduced in the scala tympani

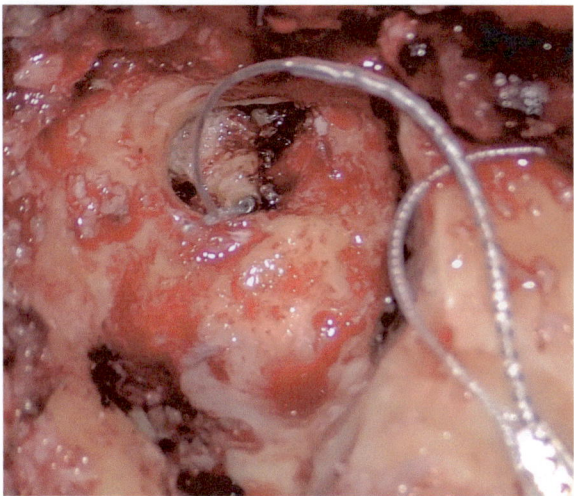

Case 8.2 *Recurrent cholesteatoma after canal wall-down tympanoplasty with no meatoplasty*

Fig. 8.8 Preoperative CT scan showing an irregular cavity with skin accumulation (white asterisk)

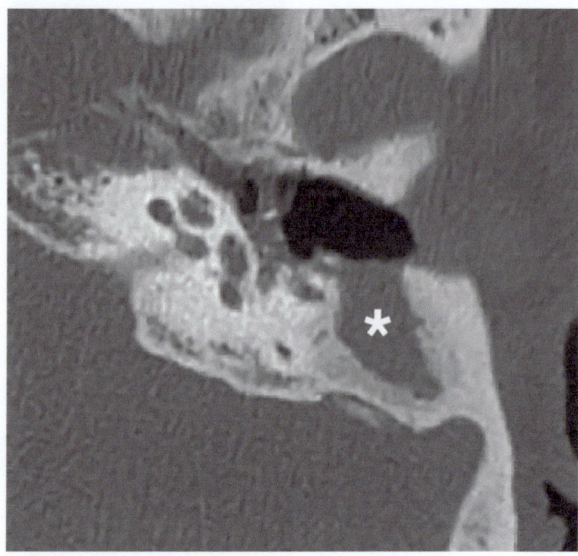

Fig. 8.9 Opening of the surgical cavity results in identification and exposure of the recurrent cholesteatoma

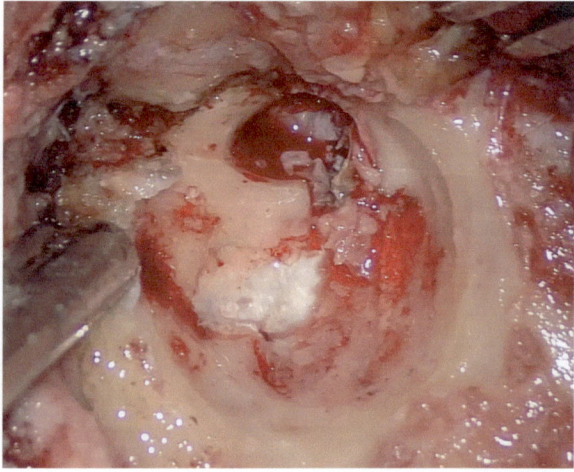

Fig. 8.10 After cholesteaoma debulking, it is possible to visualize all of the skin layering the bony cavity

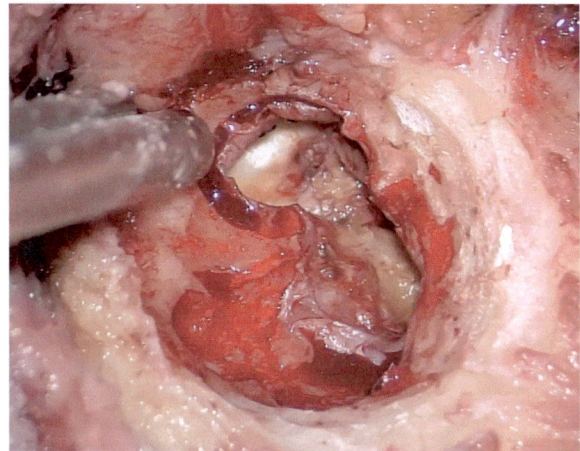

Fig. 8.11 Drilling of the bony areas previously in contact with cholesteatoma matrix is mandatory in order to further reduce the risk of residual lesion

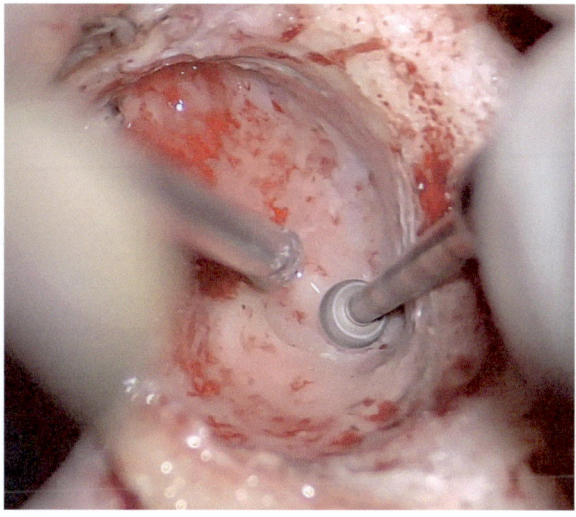

Fig. 8.12 After the cholesteatoma removal and the cavity refinements have been accomplished, the RW is opened

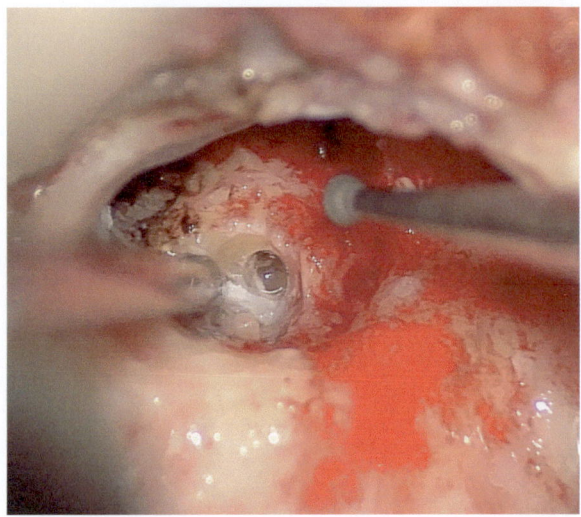

Fig. 8.13 Full array insertion is achieved through the RW

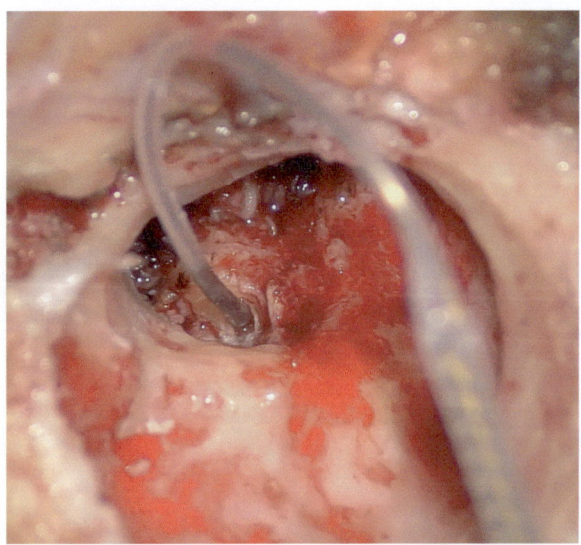

Case 8.3 Residual cholesteatoma after canal wall-up tympanoplasty

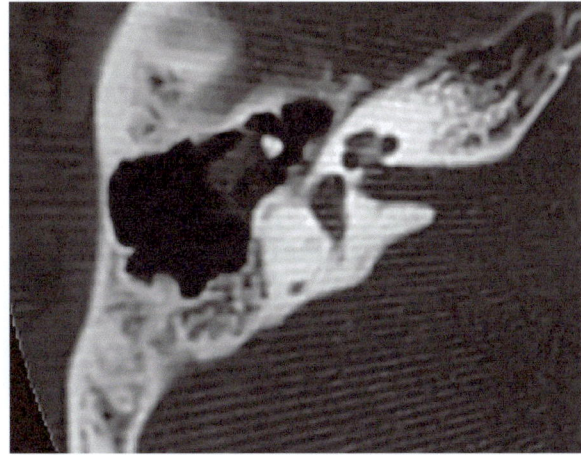

Fig. 8.14 CT showing the position of the residual cholesteatoma at the level of the aditus ad antrum

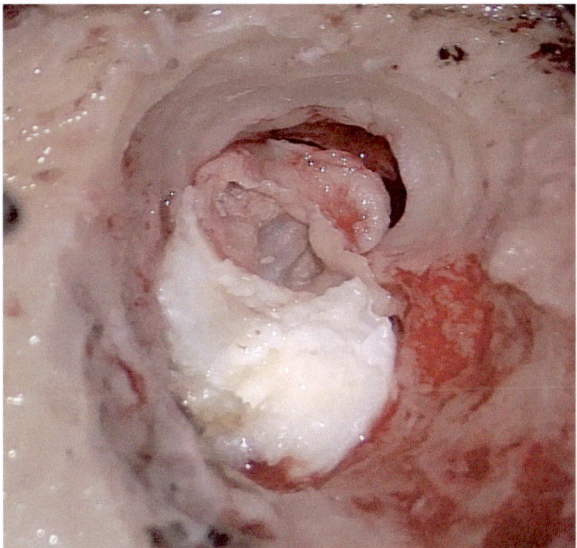

Fig. 8.15 Removal of the postero-superior wall of the EAC allows a complete control of the lesion

Fig. 8.16 Cleavage of the cholesteatoma matrix from the surrounding bony surfaces is performed with the help of a gentle elevator and a thin suction tip

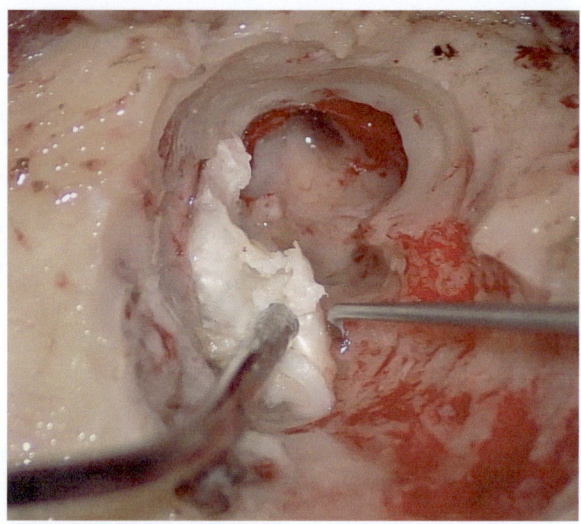

Fig. 8.17 After cholesteatoma removal, all the available pneumatization is drilled away, in order to minimize the risk of postoperative infection and cholesterol granuloma formation

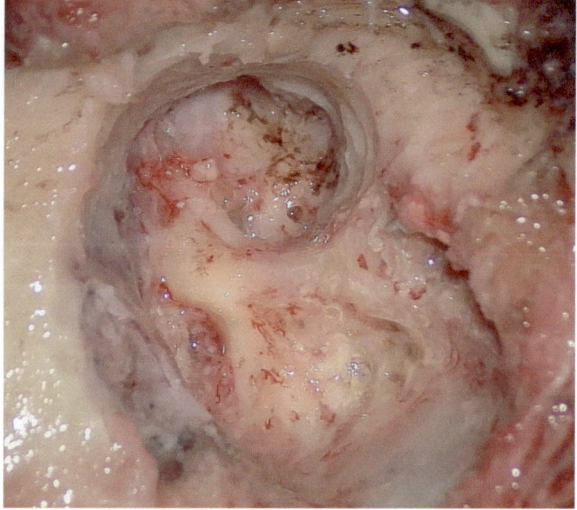

Fig. 8.18 The RW is opened in preparation for array insertion

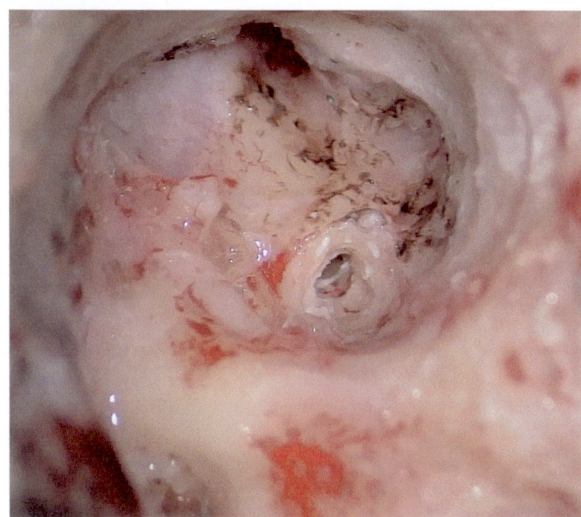

Fig. 8.19 Postoperative CT reconstructed along the cochlear axis confirms the correct and complete array insertion

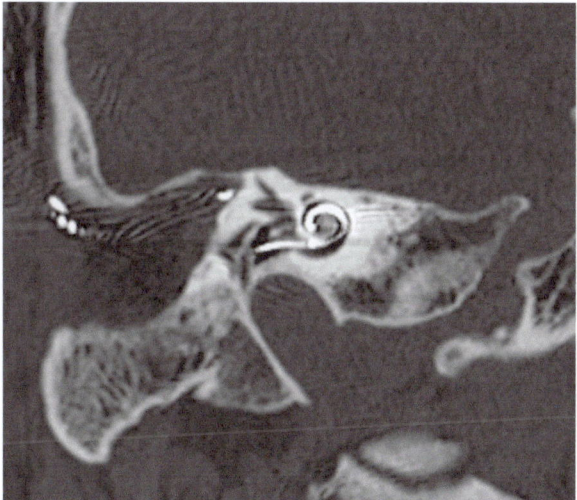

References

1. Yung M, Tono T, Olszewska E, Yamamoto Y, Sudhoff H, Sakagami M, et al. EAONO/JOS joint consensus statements on the definitions, classification and staging of middle ear cholesteatoma. J Int Adv Otology [Internet]. 2017;13(1):1–8.
2. Prasad SC, Roustan V, Piras G, Caruso A, Lauda L, Sanna M. Subtotal petrosectomy: surgical technique, indications, outcomes, and comprehensive review of literature. Laryngoscope. 2017;127(12):2833–42.
3. Pepe G, Franzini S, Guida M, Falcioni M. Subtotal petrosectomy and cochlear implantation: revision surgery. Am J Otolaryngol. 2022;43, fasc. 3:103333. https://doi.org/10.1016/j.amjoto.2021.103333.
4. Shelton C, Sheehy JL. Tympanoplasty. Laryngoscope. 1990;100(7):679–81.
5. Sanna M. Middle ear and mastoid microsurgery. Thieme; 2003.
6. Sanna M, Sunose H, Mancini F, Russo A, Taibah A. Microsurgical management of middle ear and petrous bone cholesteatoma. Thieme; 2019.
7. Más-Estellés F, Mateos-Fernández M, Carrascosa-Bisquert B, Facal de Castro F, Puchades-Román I, Morera-Pérez C. Contemporary non–echo-planar diffusion-weighted imaging of middle ear cholesteatomas. RadioGraphics. 2012;32(4):1197–213.
8. Ashraf B. Computed tomography staging of middle ear cholesteatoma. Polish J Radiol. 2015;80:328–33.

Surgical Considerations for Cochlear Implant Placement After Canal Wall-Down Tympanoplasty

9

Cochlear implantation (CI) in patients previously operated for a canal wall-down (CWD) technique should be performed selecting the subtotal petrosectomy (SP) as the safest procedure to insert a CI. In fact due to the anatomical features of the canal wall-down, the connecting cable would remain protected only by a thin layer of skin, resulting in an inevitable extrusion even in a perfectly performed cavity. As reported in the literature, previous attempts to perform some sort of reconstruction to protect the connecting cable and the array resulted in a high percentage of extrusions anyway, requiring revisions [1].

The difficulties to be managed in presence of a CWD are similar to those encountered when facing a cholesteatoma, mainly: (1) complete removal of the skin layering the cavity to avoid any risk of entrapped cholesteatoma (Figs. 9.1, 9.2, 9.3, and 9.4); (2) management of the infection (when present, take into consideration the option of a staged procedure as described in the previous chapter); (3) be prepared for the chance of intracochlear fibrosis/ossification. This latter may be the result of the infective/iatrogenic insult at the origin of the hearing loss [2]. Furthermore, some CWD cases are accompanied by a large meatoplasty, making much more difficult to properly perform the blind-sac closure of the external auditory canal (EAC). In these cases, the previous removal of the conchal cartilage makes more difficult to establish a correct dissection plane between the skin and the cartilage itself [3, 4]. As a general rule, it is easier to section the EAC even more lateral (Fig. 9.5), so that few millimeters of free skin are sufficient to be everted and sutured (Fig. 9.6). Two sutures initially positioned at the superior and inferior extremities of the sectioned skin are very helpful to pull out all the skin border to be sutured (Fig. 9.7). The Donati suture techniques are strongly recommended at this level to reduce the chances of introvertion of the skin borders (Fig. 9.8). The tragal cartilage is usually intact and can be used as a second layer (Fig. 9.9) as described in the standard SP technique in Chap. 3. It is of utmost importance to underline that in such a case, applying this surgical technique will inevitably determine a more lateral and less aesthetic closure [5, 6].

© The Author(s), under exclusive license to Springer Nature
Switzerland AG 2025
M. Falcioni et al., *Cochlear Implant - Rare and Difficult Cases*,
https://doi.org/10.1007/978-3-032-02323-0_9

Case 9.1 Patient treated with a previous canal wall-down

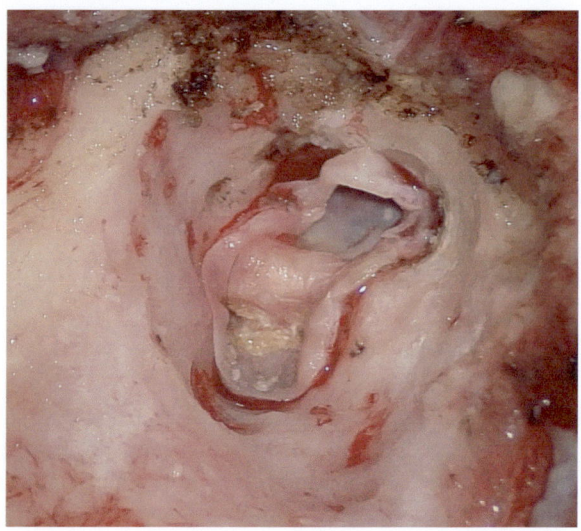

Fig. 9.1 The initial appearance of the previous cavity

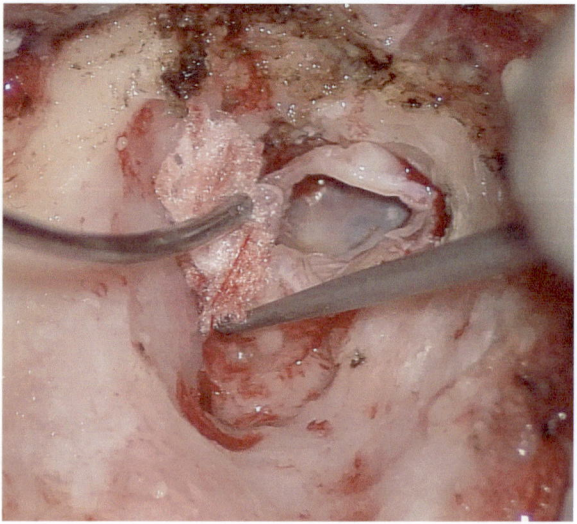

Fig. 9.2 Careful en-blok dissection of the skin layering the cavity reduces the risk of leaving some remnants

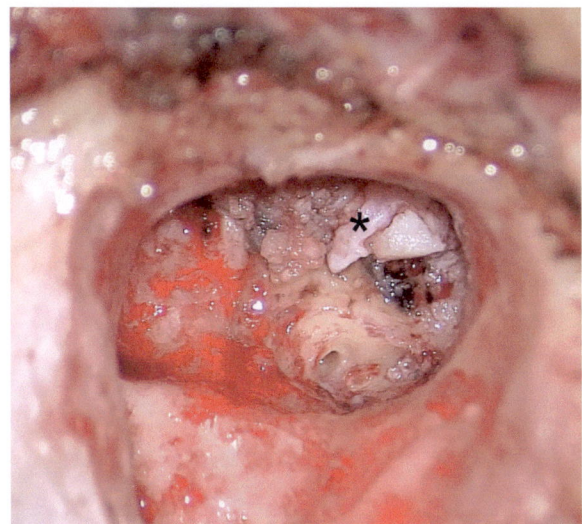

Fig. 9.3 After cleaning and coagulation of the mucosa of the middle ear cleft, the round window is clearly exposed. The Eustachian tube orifice has already been plugged with muscle and cartilage (black asterisk) and the RW opened and prepared for array insertion

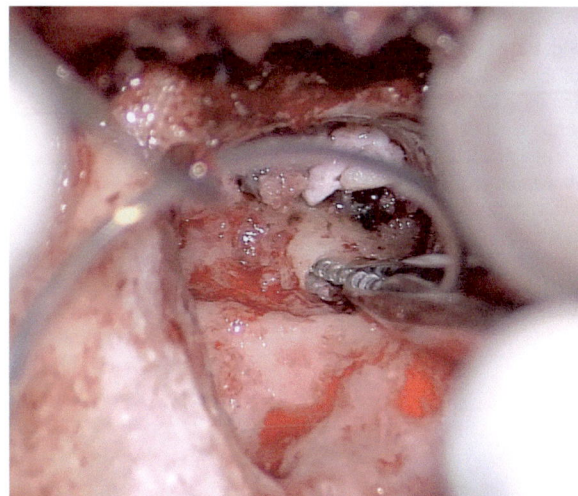

Fig. 9.4 The array is correctly inserted into the cochlear lumen

Case 9.2 Patient treated with a previous canal wall-down with a large meatoplasty

Fig. 9.5 The EAC and the huge meatoplasty has been transected very laterally; the pinna is anteriorly reflected to facilitate the dissection of the skin from the cartilage

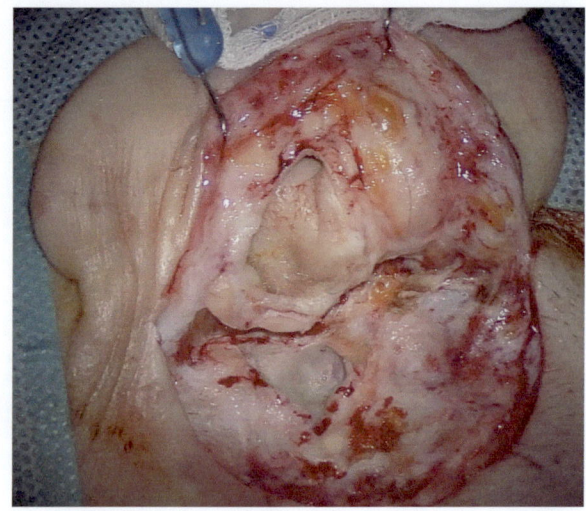

Fig. 9.6 The skin borders of the meatoplasty are only freed for a few millimeters at the level of the conchal cartilage, taking care not to damage them. The skin layering the tragal cartilage is managed as in the standard EAC closure described in Chap 2

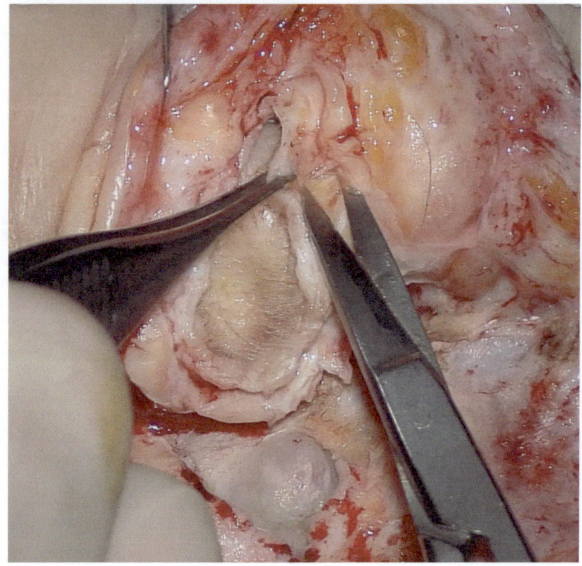

Fig. 9.7 Two sutures are positioned at the superior and inferior corners of the sectioned skin, in order to make easier the eversion and suture of the central areas

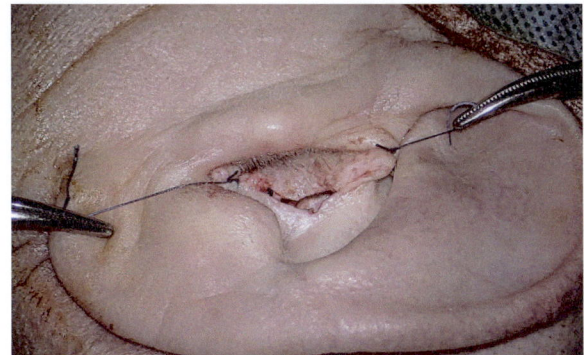

Fig. 9.8 The skin borders are completely sealed. Adopting the Donati suture technique decreases the chances of skin introflection and entrapment

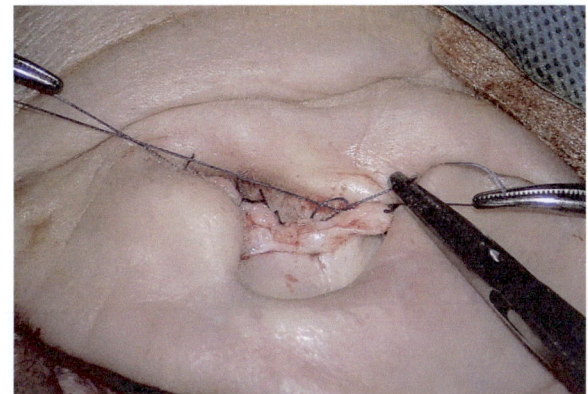

Fig. 9.9 Since the tragal cartilage is usually intact in a meatoplasty, the second layer closure is performed in the standard modality, posteriorly reflecting the cartilage itself and suturing this latter to the subcutaneous tissue

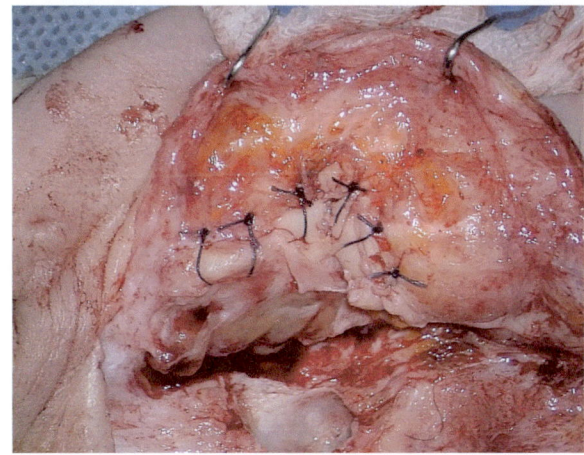

References

1. Issing PR, et al. Cochlear implantation in patients with chronic otitis: Indications for subtotal petrosectomy and obliteration of the Middle Ear. Skull Base. 1998;8(03):127–31. https://doi.org/10.1055/s-2008-1058571.
2. Canzano F, Di Lella F, Guida M, Pasanisi E, Govoni M, Falcioni M. Revision cochlear implant surgery for clinical reasons. Acta Otorhinolaryngologica Italica [Internet]. 2023. [cited 2023 Apr 23];43(1):65–73.
3. Hunter JB, O'Connell BP, Wanna GB. Systematic review and meta-analysis of surgical complications following cochlear implantation in canal wall down mastoid cavities. Otolaryngol Head Neck Surg. 2016;155(4):555–63.
4. Gao S, Jiang Y, Wang GJ, Li BC, Yuan YY, Gao B, et al. Cochlear implantation in patients with canal wall down mastoidectomy cavities. Acta Oto-Laryngologica. 2018;138(11):993–7.
5. Coker NJ, Jenkins HA, Fisch U. Obliteration of the middle ear and mastoid cleft in subtotal petrosectomy: indications, technique, and results. Ann Otol Rhinol Laryngol. 1986;95(1):5–11. https://doi.org/10.1177/000348948609500102.
6. Sanna M. Surgery for Cochlear and other auditory implants, 2015. Stuttgart: Thieme; 2015.

Cochlear Implants in Ear Malformations: Surgical Strategy

10

Inner ear malformation represents one of the most challenging chapters in hearing rehabilitation and otologic surgery [1]. Most of these abnormalities are due to an interruption of the embryological development of the ear during the first trimester of pregnancy. The causes are numerous; among the most common we can find autosomal dominant or recessive genetic disease, external teratogenic factors, or radiation exposure. There are two groups of malformations: membranous inner ear malformations and bony labyrinth malformations. Approximately, 80% of congenital hearing loss are due to membranous malformations; no bony deformities are associated and visible at radiological evaluation. These patients are candidates to cochlear implantation and the surgery is performed through a standard approach [2]. The residual 20% of the congenital hearing loss have osseous labyrinth malformations that can be radiologically visualized by computed tomography (CT) scan and magnetic resonance imaging (MRI) (Figs. 10.1, 10.2, 10.3, 10.4, and 10.5). Cochlear nerve malformations are often associated with bony abnormalities of the inner ear and should be carefully investigated for the potential to deeply influence the final result. Malformations may be confined to the inner ear or combined with others in different areas of the body; in this case, the patients are classified as "syndromic" (Usher's syndrome, Alport's syndrome, CHARGE (Figs. 10.13, 10.14, 10.15, 10.16, 10.17, 10.18, 10.19, 10.20, and 10.21), Down syndrome, BOR, Figs. 10.22, 10.23, 10.24, 10.25, and 10.26), Pendred syndrome, Klippel-Feil syndrome, etc.) [3–7].

A wide range of bony malformations have been described, from complete absence of the cochlea to a mild enlargement of the vestibule. The Sennaroglu classification is presently the most updated and adopted and includes a large variety of malformations.[1] Some of them are not candidates for CI surgery, because there is no available cochlear lumen to insert any array. Luckily the majority of the cases are treatable with cochlear implantation, often through the standard approach, taking care to select an array that can match the shape of the cochlea and the supposed distribution of the sensorial epithelium [2].

However, some malformations may present some surgical difficulties to be managed. The most important problem is represented by the risk of cerebrospinal fluid (CSF) leak during or even after the surgery. This occurs in the presence of bony deformities at the level of the cochlear aperture and/or the modiolus (Fig. 10.6); the inner ear is connected with the subarachnoid space, and opening of the cochleostomy inevitably results in a CSF leak (Figs. 10.6, 10.7, 10.8, 10.9, 10.10, 10.11, and 10.12). Different solutions have been proposed, but the safest one remains the performance of a subtotal petrosectomy (SP) [8]. In this case, in addition to the blockage of the cochleostomy, the obliteration of the Eustachian tube works as a second barrier against the leak, and the fat filling the surgical cavity as a third barrier. In rare case of large communication between the inner ear and the internal auditory canal (IAC), an intraoperative radiological evaluation is strongly advised to immediately detect an accidental array insertion into the IAC.

When dealing with such cases, additional difficulties are represented by the fact that all the young patients are non-cooperating; and as a consequence, the stimulation map should be built only in agreement with the neural responses.

Sometimes, especially in syndromic patient, inner ear malformations are combined with middle ear and temporal bone abnormalities. These include vascular malformations, absence of the round and/or oval window, and anomalous route of the facial nerve. More rarely, these malformations are present in the absence of inner ear malformations radiologically visible. The absence of the common landmarks adopted for otologic surgery represents an extremely dangerous situation; as a consequence, these cases must be treated in referral otologic centers. The SP represents the best surgical option even for the majority of these patients, due to the large surgical field and the possibility to better identify the few available landmarks.

Case 10.1 *Patient affected by a common cavity. The main difficulty is represented by the impossibility to know the position of what remains of the sensorial epithelium along the lateral surface of the round cavity. In such a situation, sound detection is the only realistic expectation.*

10 Cochlear Implants in Ear Malformations: Surgical Strategy

Fig. 10.1 MRI shows bilateral single cystic cavity with no separation between cochlear and vestibular compartments and complete absence of the modiolus, usually hosting the terminal cochlear nerve fibers

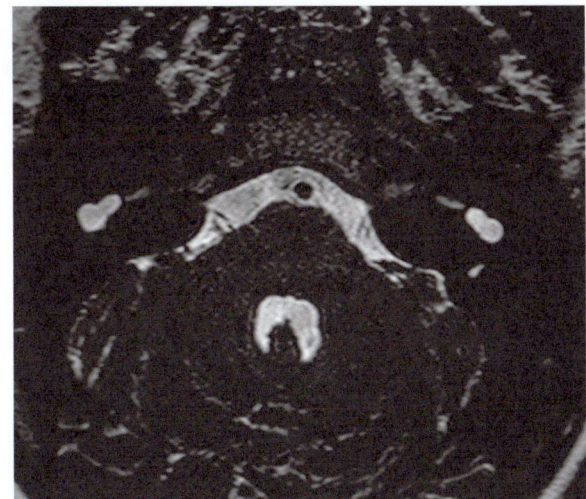

Fig. 10.2 A slit (white arrow) has been opened along the direction of the outline of the rudimental lateral semicircular canal in order to access the inner ear cavity

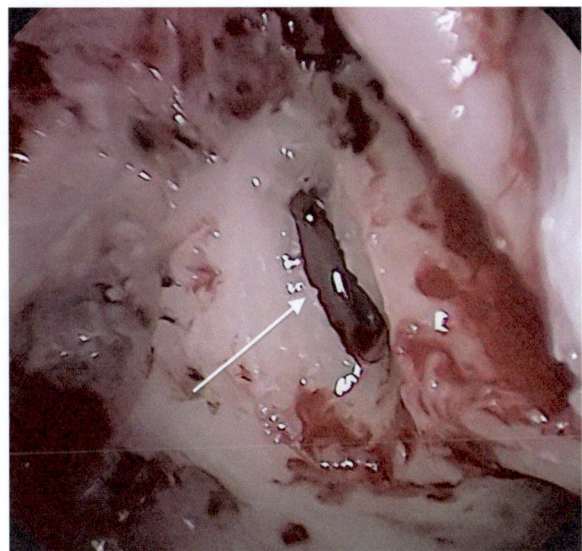

Fig. 10.3 A loop of a full-banded array has been inserted into the slit, trying to maximize the contact surface with the lateral wall of the cavity, the theoretical location of the sensorineural epitelium. The tip of the array is visible emerging from the slit

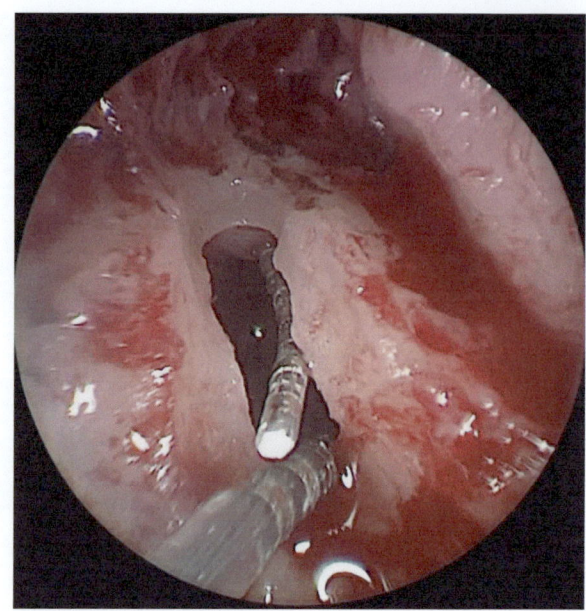

Fig. 10.4 Postoperative X-ray showing the loop of the array (white arrow) into the cavity

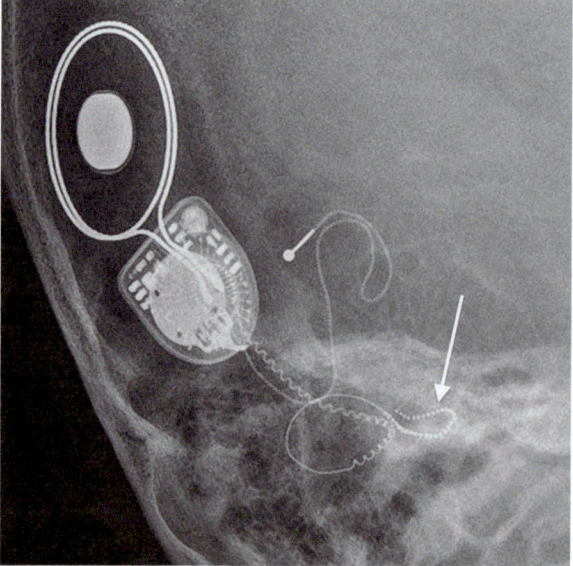

10 Cochlear Implants in Ear Malformations: Surgical Strategy

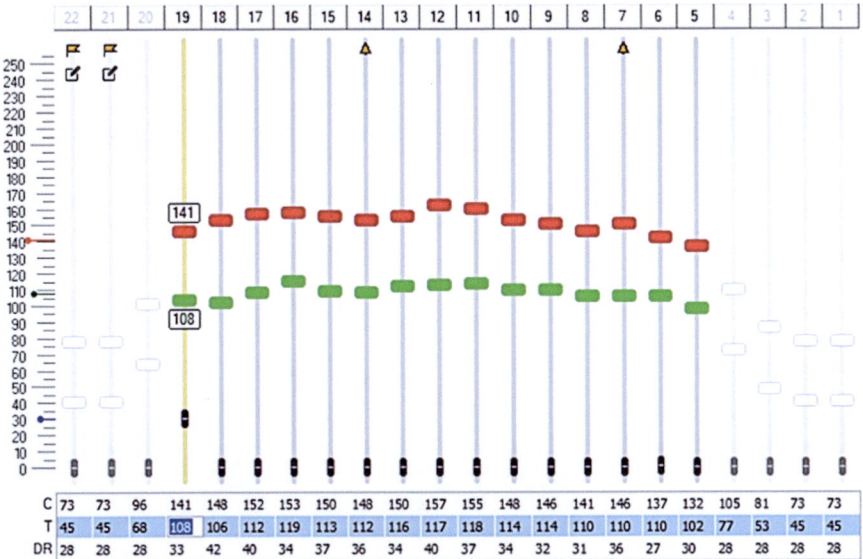

Fig. 10.5 In agreement with the intraoperative images, the basal (1–4) and apical (20–22) electrodes result outside the cavity and, as a consequence, have not been activated. The stimulation levels exceed the standard range (pursuit 62). The tonotopicity must be artificially built and, of course, the action potential is not recorded in any electrode

Case 10.2 *Patient affected by an incomplete partition type 2. The main difficulty is represented by the high risk of CSF leak and an SP is selected accordingly. A full-banded array is preferred because of the absence of the superior portion of the modiolus.*

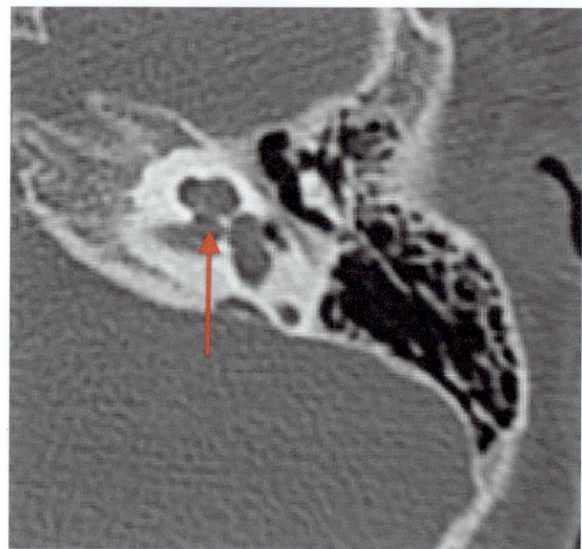

Fig. 10.6 Axial CT showing the fusion of the middle and apical turns of the cochlea with no modiolus and interscalar septa at this level. Note the wide communication between the cochlea and the fundus of the internal auditory canal (red arrow)

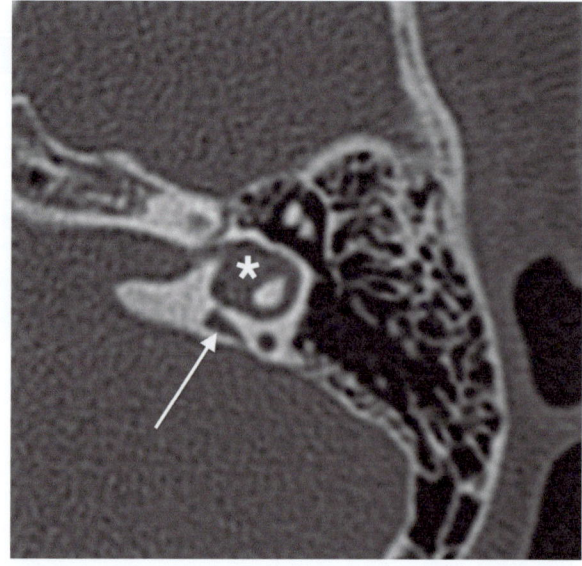

Fig. 10.7 A superior section of the same CT allows identification of the large vestibule (white asterisk) and the enlarged vestibular aqueduct (white arrow), confirming the diagnosis of incomplete partition type II

10 Cochlear Implants in Ear Malformations: Surgical Strategy

Fig. 10.8 The SP has been accomplished; a small RW niche is visualized. A small cochleostomy is created to facilitate its packing to stop/reduce the leakage at the end of the procedure

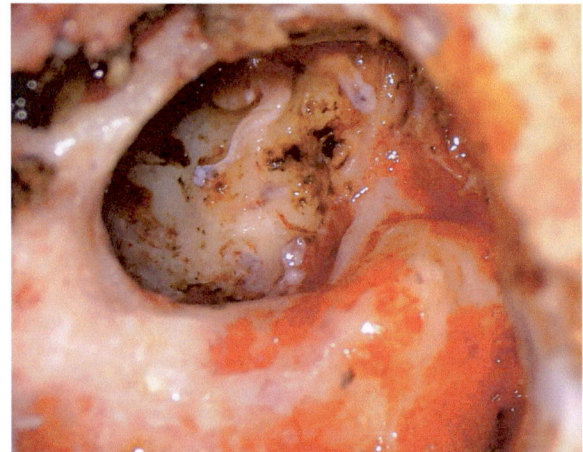

Fig. 10.9 A total insertion of the full-banded array is achieved

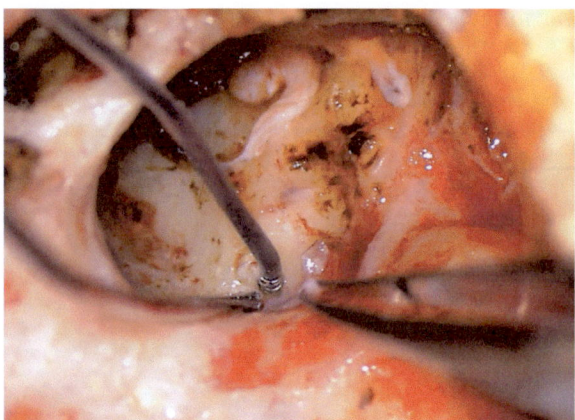

Fig. 10.10 In spite of the tissue positioned all around the entrance of the array into the cochleostomy, some leak is still present, slowly filling the surgical cavity. This underlines the importance of the second and third barriers represented by the obliteration of the Eustachian tube orifice and the fat filling the surgical cavity

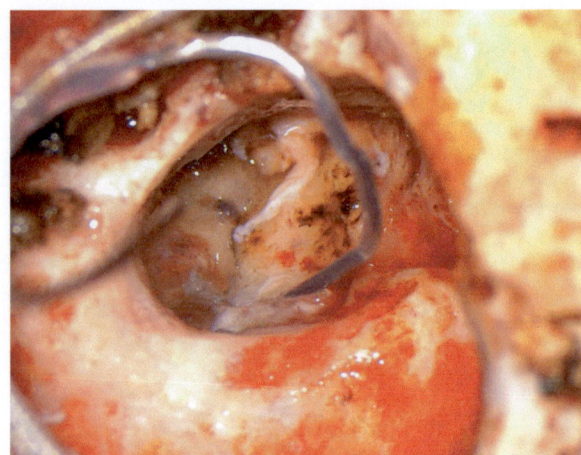

Fig. 10.11 Postoperative CT scan showing the correct position of the array on the lateral wall of the middle turn

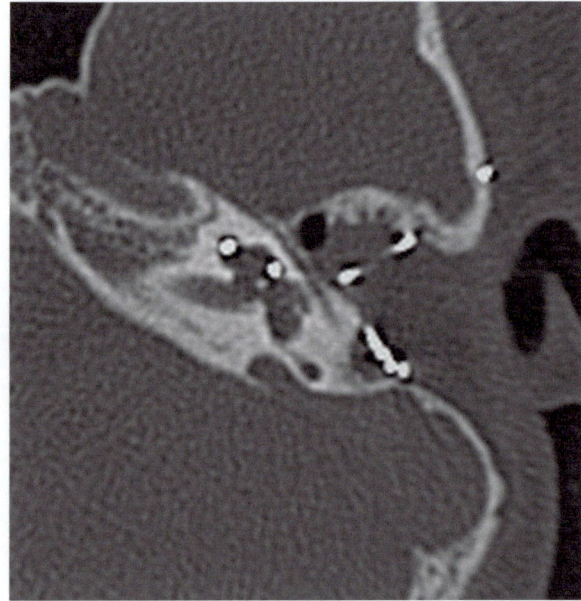

10 Cochlear Implants in Ear Malformations: Surgical Strategy

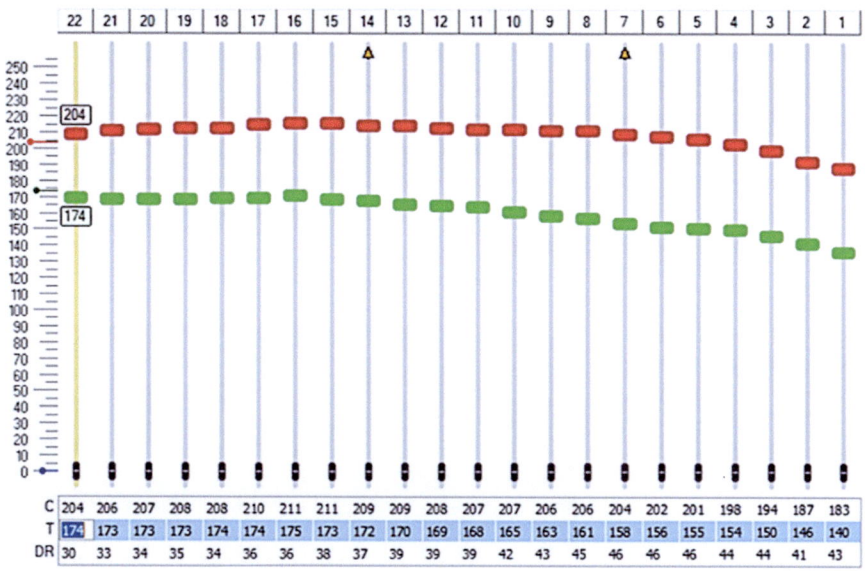

Fig. 10.12 Post-operatively the patient required stimulation levels higher than the standard range. However, they resulted sufficient to obtain open set recognition performances

Case 10.3 *Patient affected by a CHARGE syndrome, in which the cochlea is often well developed while the most common inner ear anomalies are represented by the absence of the lateral semicircular canal and the windows. In this specific case, the main difficulties are represented by vascular anomalies into the mastoid and the absence of the round window. A draining ear, consequence of an atelectatic tympanic membrane, made the case even more demanding. Due to the impossibility to access the mastoid, an enlarged canalplasty combined with a blindsac closure of the EAC was the approach selected.*

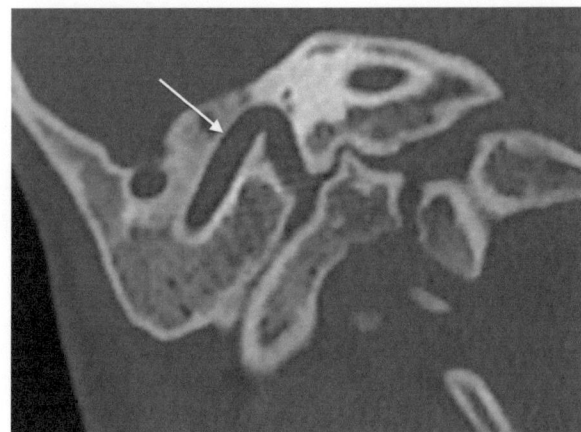

Fig. 10.13 Preoperative coronal CT; huge venous vessels (white arrow) run through a sclerotic mastoid

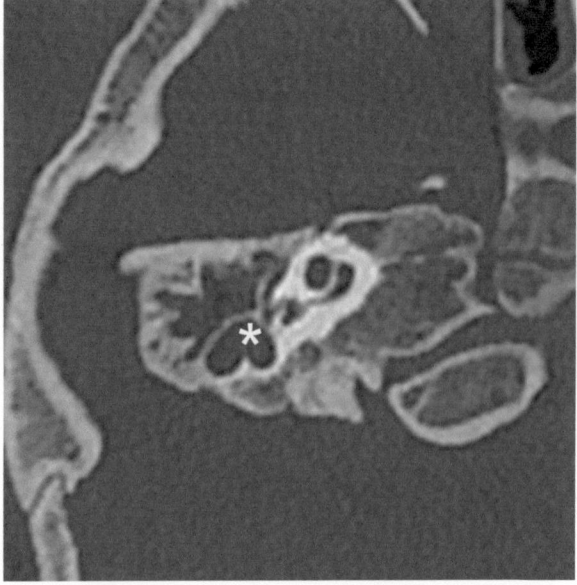

Fig. 10.14 The vascular malformations (white asterisk) reach the posterior border of the cochlea, in the area of the RW

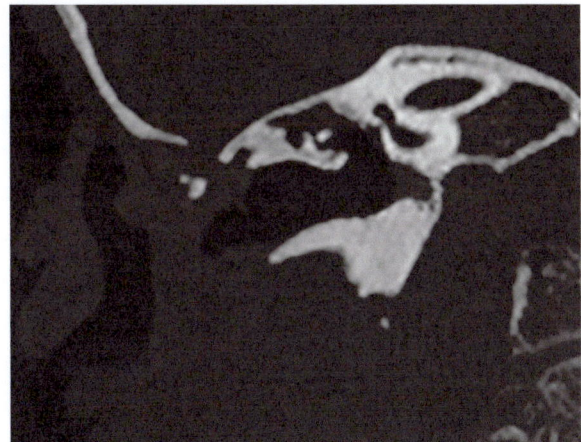

Fig. 10.15 CT, coronal view. The lateral semicircular canal is not developed, a common finding in CHARGE syndrome, and the absence of the round window is confirmed as well. A previous standard approach had already been attempted in another center and aborted intraoperatively

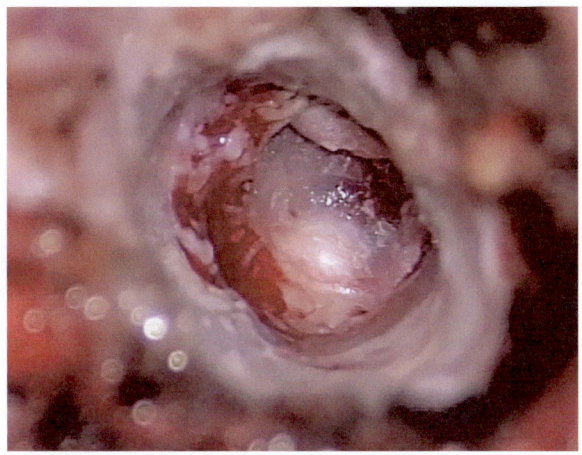

Fig. 10.16 Intraoperatively an atelectatic tympanic membrane was visualized after surgical enlargement of a very narrow EAC. The patient was affected by recurrent ear discharge

Fig. 10.17 Following a careful removal of the EAC skin, the tympanic membrane, malleus, and incus, because of the absence of the round window, a promontorial drilling is started inferiorly to the stapes (white arrow)

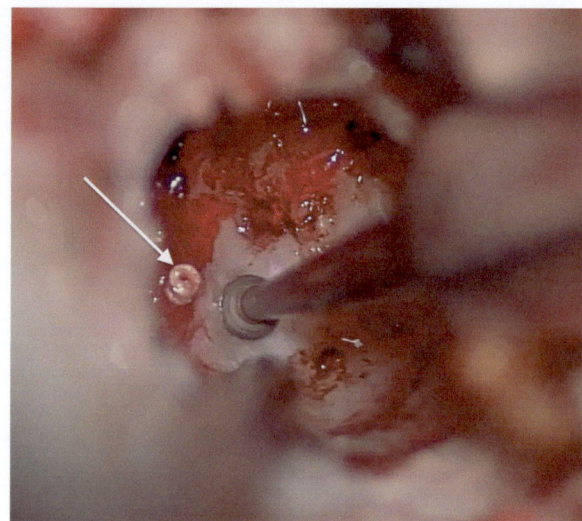

Fig. 10.18 The final cochleostomy (white arrow) is then performed

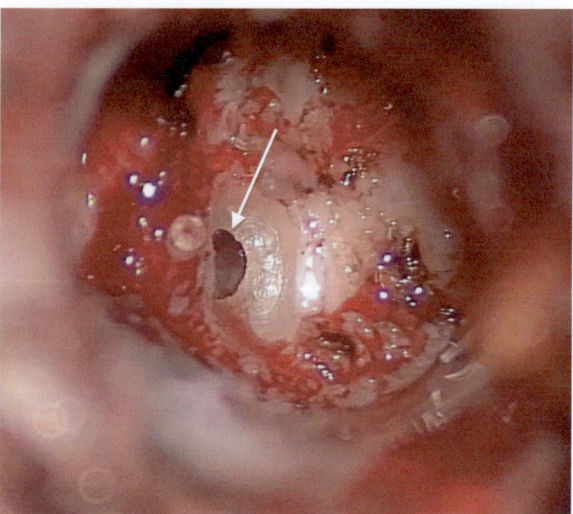

Fig. 10.19 After packing of the Eustachian tube orifice, a full array insertion is achieved

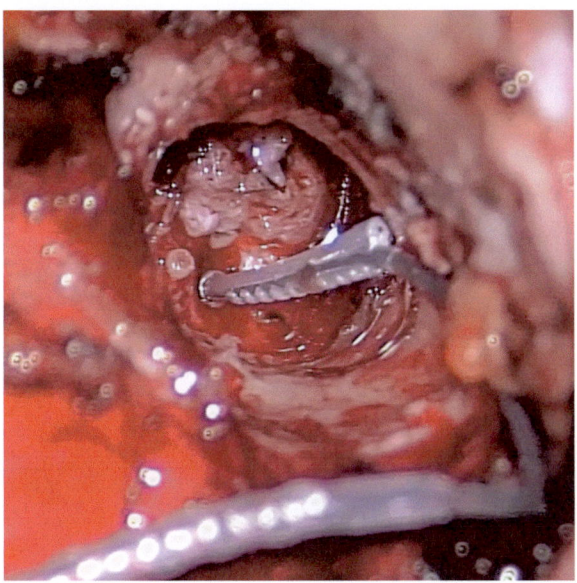

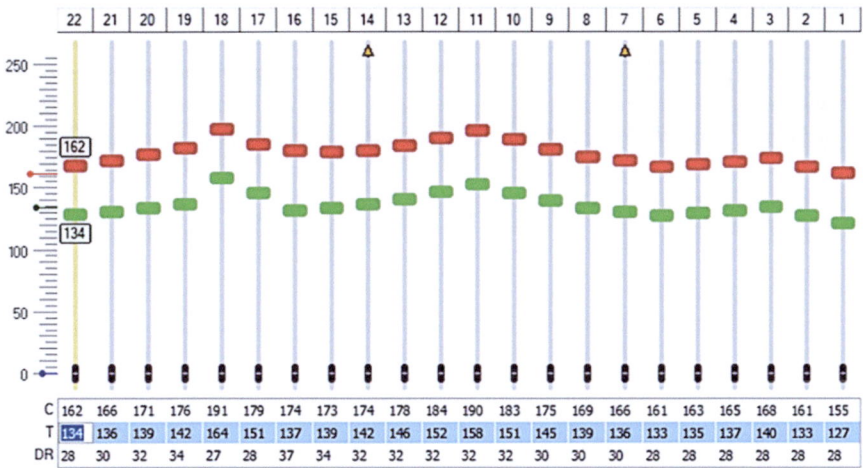

Fig. 10.20 Even in this case, the level of stimulation for every single electrode was determined only on the base of the neural responses

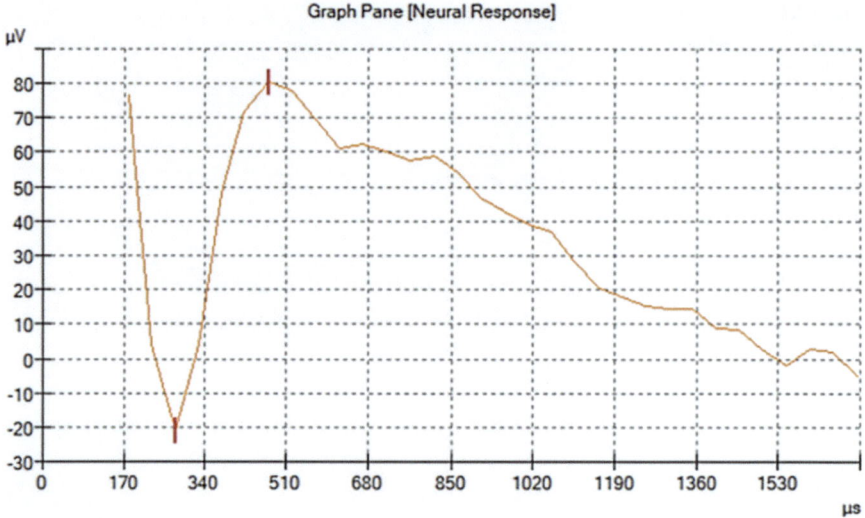

Fig. 10.21 All the electrodes have been activated with a good neural depolarization

Case 10.4 *Patient affected by a BOR (Branchio-Oto-Renal) syndrome, in which a hypoplastic cochlea was present, as well as a large vestibular aqueduct. However, the surgical difficulties were not related to the inner ear malformations, but to the anomalies of the middle ear and temporal bone, mainly the anomalous route of the facial nerve (with the tympanic portion not radiologically visible on the CT scan) and the very low running dura of the middle cranial fossa. Even if not mandatory, SP was selected to better identify and control the anatomical landmarks.*

10 Cochlear Implants in Ear Malformations: Surgical Strategy

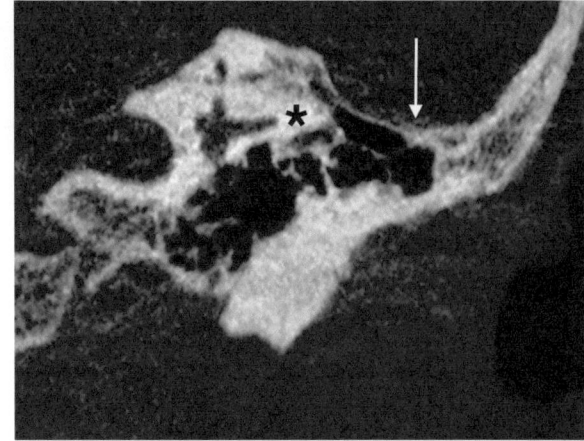

Fig. 10.22 CT scan, coronal view; a very low middle cranial fossa (white arrows) dura runs inferior to the level of the lateral semicircular canal (black asterisk). This makes the angle of the approach to the area of the posterior tympanotomy very uncomfortable

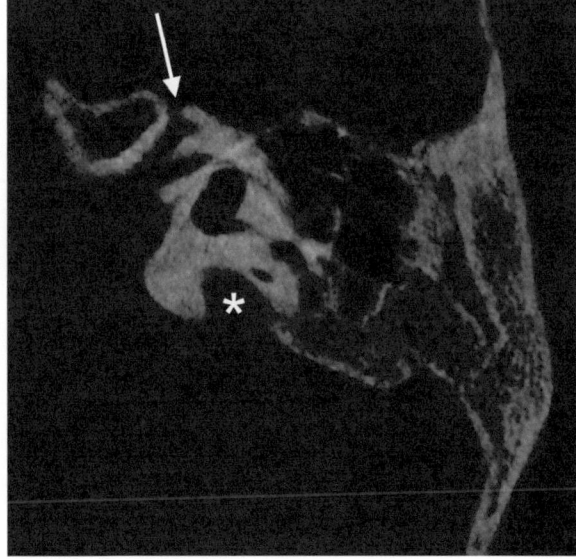

Fig. 10.23 CT scan, axial view; the labyrinthine portion of the facial nerve (white arrow) follows an anterior route. The vestibular aqueduct (white asterisk) appears enlarged

Fig. 10.24 CT scan, axial view; the middle and apical turn of the cochlea appear hypoplastic (white arrow)

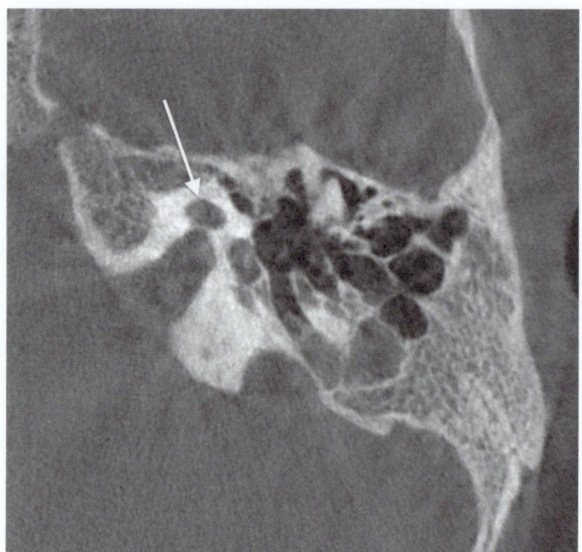

Fig. 10.25 After completing the initial steps of the SP, the facial nerve (white asterisk) was easily identified, in the standard position. In spite of the large working room provided by the SP, due to the lower middle cranial fossa dura, the bony work was accomplished through an uncomfortable inferior-to-superior angle. Note the large stapedial muscle (black asterisk)

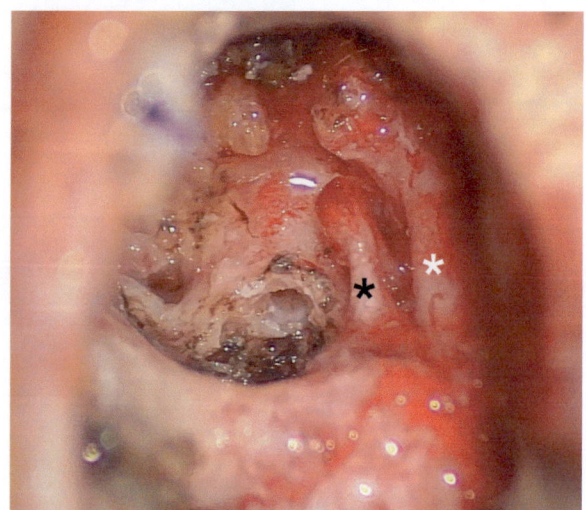

Fig. 10.26 In spite of the short cochlea, the array was completely inserted into the lumen

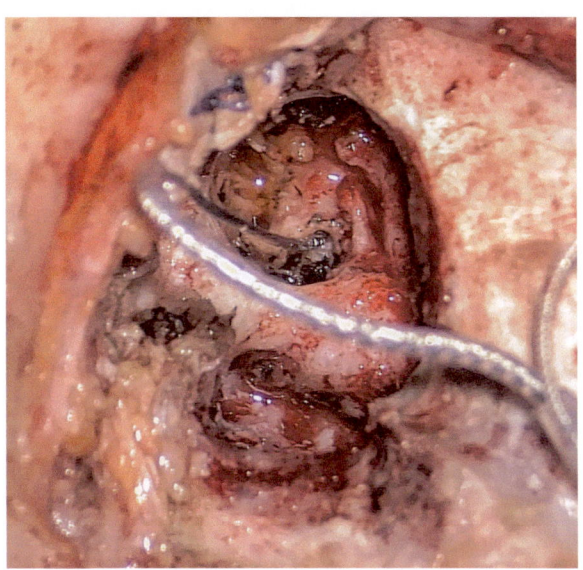

References

1. Sennaroğlu L, Demir Bajin M. Classification and current management of inner ear malformations. Balkan Med J [Internet]. 2017;34(5):397–411.
2. Farhood Z, Nguyen SA, Miller SC, Holcomb MA, Meyer TA, Rizk HG. Cochlear implantation in inner ear malformations: systematic review of speech perception outcomes and intraoperative findings. Otolaryngol Head Neck Surg. 2017;156(5):783–93.
3. Sanna M. Surgery for cochlear and other auditory implants, 2015. Stuttgart: Thieme; 2015.
4. Bauer PW, Wippold FJ II, Goldin J, Lusk RP. Cochlear implantation in children with CHARGE association. Arch Otolaryngol Head Neck Surg. 2002;128(9):1013.
5. Song MH, Kwon TJ, Kim HR, Jeon JH, Baek JI, Lee WS, et al. Mutational analysis of EYA1, SIX1 and SIX5 genes and strategies for management of hearing loss in patients with BOR/BO syndrome. PLoS One [Internet]. 2013. [cited 2025 Feb 2];8(6):e67236–6.
6. Kontorinis G, Lenarz T, Lesinski-Schiedat A, Neuburger J. Cochlear implantation in Pendred syndrome. Cochlear Implants Int. 2011;12(3):157–63.
7. Loundon N, Marlin S, Busquet D, Denoyelle F, Roger G, Renaud F, et al. Usher syndrome and cochlear implantation. Otol Neurotol. 2003;24(2):216–21.
8. Coker NJ, Jenkins HA, Fisch U. Obliteration of the middle ear and mastoid cleft in subtotal petrosectomy: indications, technique, and results. Ann Otol Rhinol Laryngol. 1986;95(1):5–11. https://doi.org/10.1177/000348948609500102.

Temporal Bone Fractures and Otic Capsule Involvement: Surgical Tips in Cochlear Implantation

11

Temporal bone fractures crossing the otic capsule unavoidably implicate a dead ear; in order to attempt an hearing rehabilitation in such ears with a CI, the surgeons should be aware of the possibility of facing many difficulties [1].

First, as a result of the trauma, the patient usually is affected by additional severe medical problems, often life-threatening, and so the timing of otological evaluation is frequently delayed, sometimes even of a few months [2].

This may induce a cochlear ossification (Figs. 11.4 and 11.5), especially when the fracture line crosses the cochlea itself, making the implantation difficult if still possible (Fig. 11.11). Another problem is represented by the fact that the otic capsule never heals with new bone formation; the site of the fracture is filled by fibrous tissue, representing a theoretical route for intracranial infection even many years after the trauma [3]. This requires a solution that may guarantee the isolation of the fracture line from the external environment. Facial nerve lesions often are combined with the dead ear and may require a grafting during the same surgery. The worst fractures may show a dislocation of the bony fragments, resulting in an absence of reliable landmarks during surgery (Figs. 11.10, 11.11, 11.12, 11.13, 11.14, 11.15, 11.16, 11.17, 11.18, and 11.19). An additional complications is sometime represented by concomitant traumas at the level of the tympanic membrane and/or the external auditory canal (Fig. 11.12) [4]. As a consequence, the patient can develop a chronic otitis/cholesteatoma, sometimes immediately, in other cases in the long run (see Chap. 13).

For all these reasons, the majority of the fractures are better treated through the SP [5]. The approach is helpful in facing all the aforementioned difficulties, offering a better chance of promontorium drill-out in case of ossification (Fig. 11.1, 11.2, 11.3, 11.4, 11.5, 11.6, 11.7, 11.8, and 11.9), eliminating forever the risk of an intracranial infection (even not related to the implant), managing the facial nerve when required and allowing the surgeon to have a better anatomical control of the surgical field [6].

Hearing rehabilitation with cochlear implantation in patients following temporal bone trauma strongly depends on the spiral ganglion cells population still available for stimulation. The promontory test may be extremely helpful to evaluate this parameter and predict the postoperative performances. In the author's experience, a good result of the promontory test strongly suggests the potential for the patient to reach a satisfactory result.

The appropriate electrophysiological stimulation strategy may take into consideration the neural pool, the number of active electrodes, the site of anatomical lesion, as well as the presence of some amount of cochlear ossification, almost inevitably present. The possibility of having an undesired facial nerve stimulation should be taken into consideration, as already described in otosclerosis chapter 5.

Case 11.1 *Temporal bone fracture with partial ossification. At another center, the patient was considered not a good candidate for a CI and underwent an ABI. With only 5 electrodes working and limited acoustic benefit, the ABI was abandoned in 2 years. After some time and a new radiological and audiological evaluation, the option of a CI was reconsidered. In particular, the promontory test showed a good neural activity, especially regarding the sequential and temporal discrimination. 1 year after the CI, the patient reached 100% of words and sentences recognition in open set.*

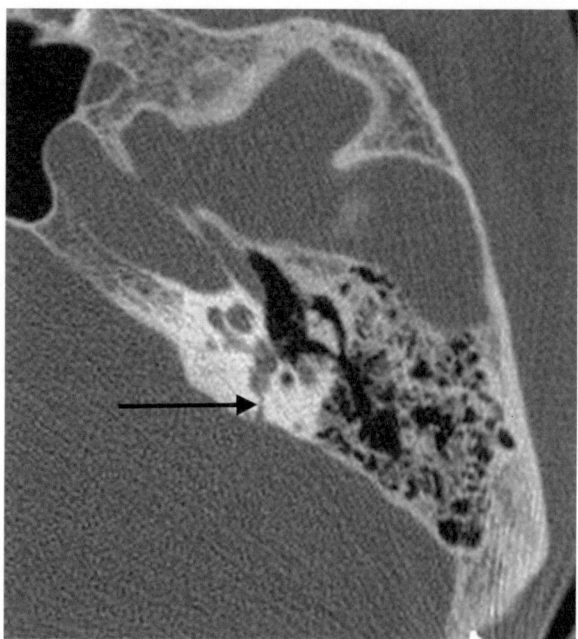

Fig. 11.1 Preoperative axial CT showing the fracture line (black arrow) crossing the vestibule

Fig. 11.2 Initial view of the surgical field after the SP has been completed. Note the fibrotic tissue (black asterisk) present at the level of the OW and RW area

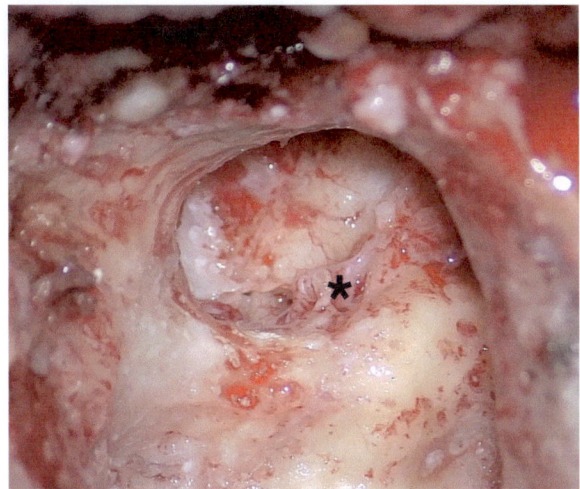

Fig. 11.3 Once the fibrotic tissues has been removed, the fracture line (black arrow) is clearly visualized, running in between the OW and the RW

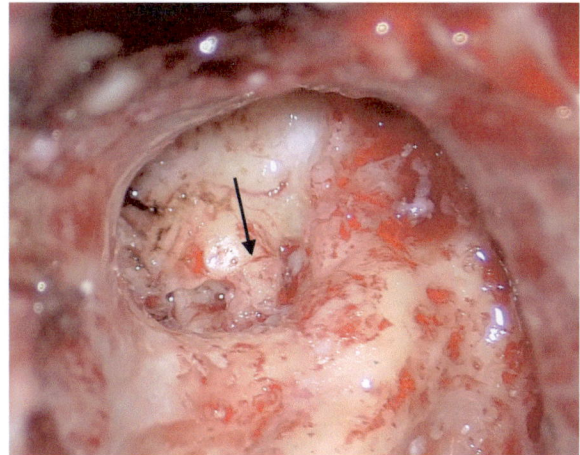

Fig. 11.4 The presence of some ossification at the level of the RW (black arrow) requires a basal turn drill-out to identify a cochlear lumen

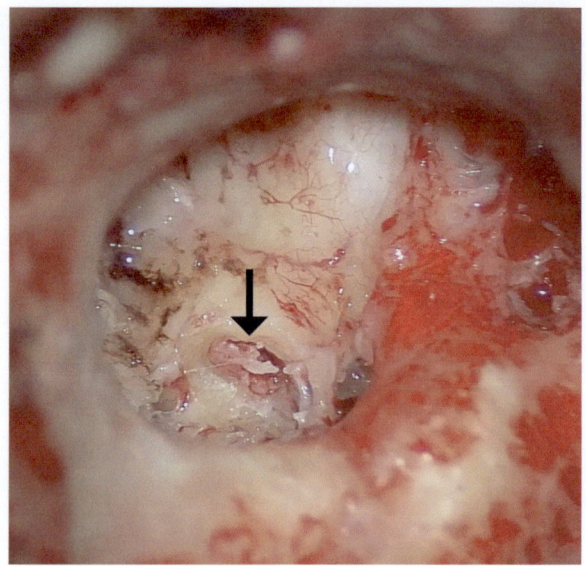

Fig. 11.5 The cleaning of the cochleostomy has been completed and the cochlea is ready for implantation

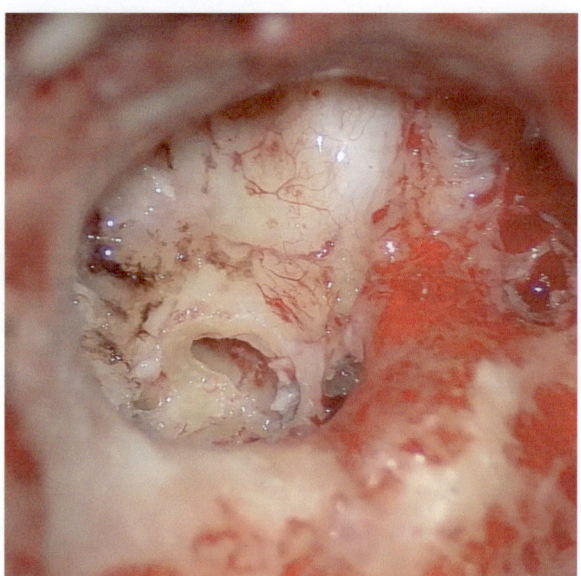

Fig. 11.6 Postoperative axial CT showing the correct position of the array in the cochlea

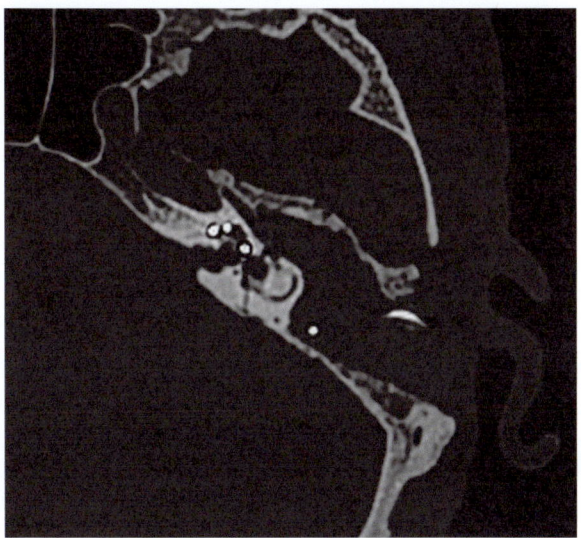

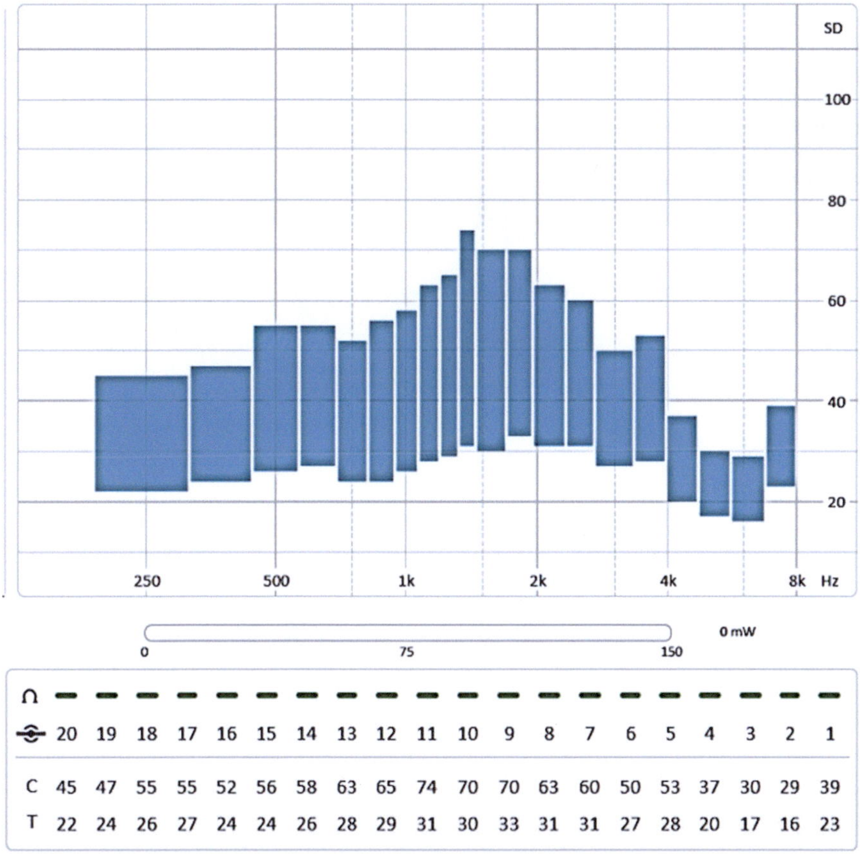

SD
100
80
60
40
20
250
500
1k
2k
4k
8k
Hz
0 mW
0
75
150
20 19 18 17 16 15 14 13 12 11 10 9 8 7 6 5 4 3 2 1
C 45 47 55 55 52 56 58 63 65 74 70 70 63 60 50 53 37 30 29 39
T 22 24 26 27 24 24 26 28 29 31 30 33 31 31 27 28 20 17 16 23

Fig. 11.7 All the electrodes have been positively activated with stimulation levels within the normal range. These parameters confirmed the positive data obtained with the preoperative promontory test

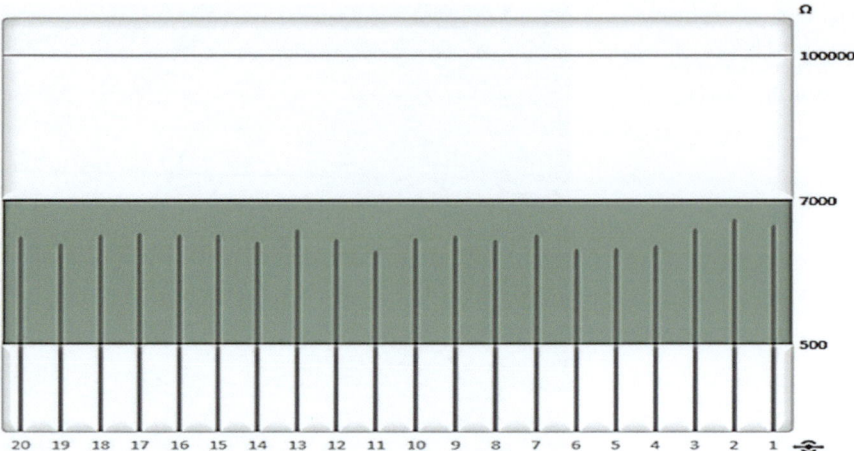

Fig. 11.8 The impedences of all the electrodes are in the standard range, confirming the absence of abnormalities of the cochlear lumen once overcome the initial ossification at the level of the trauma (the round window area)

Fig. 11.9 The EABR shows a good neural conduction till the brainstem, confirming the integrity of the cochlear nuclei even after the ABI

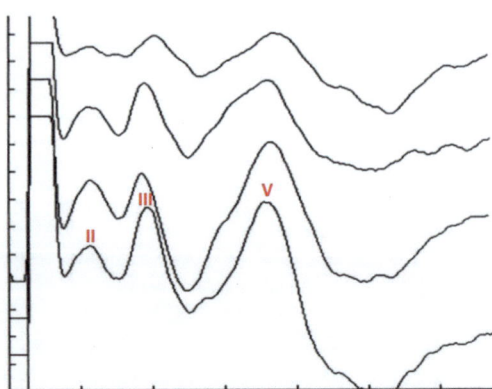

Case 11.2 Bilateral temporal bone fractures with displacement of the bony fragments and complete cochlear ossification on the right side. SP with cochlear implantation in the left side, a discharging ear due to post-traumatic retraction pocket.

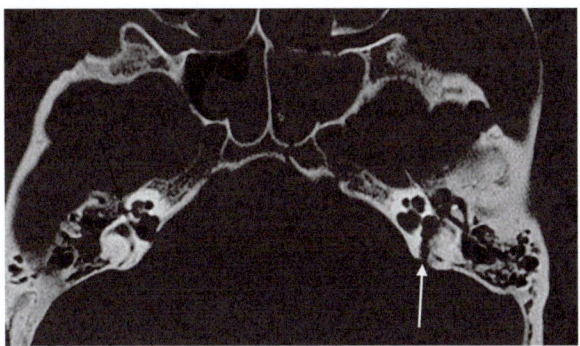

Fig. 11.10 Temporal bone CT immediately after the trauma, showing bilateral temporal bone fractures. On the right side, the fracture line (black arrow) crosses the cochlea entering the internal auditory canal (note the air bubbles in both the structures). On the left side, the fracture line (white arrow) crosses the vestibule, leaving a wide gap between the bony fragments. The patient suffered a lot of additional traumas (see another fracture at the level of the clivus/sphenoid sinus) and spent 3 months in the intensive care unit

Fig. 11.11 Preoperative MRI, 3 months after the trauma, shows a complete absence of fluid in the right cochlea (red arrow). On the contrary, the intracochlear fluids are still present on the left side (green arrow)

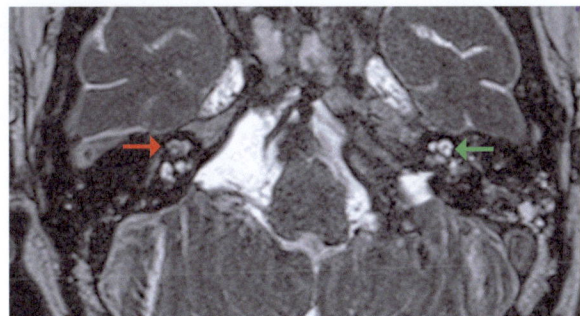

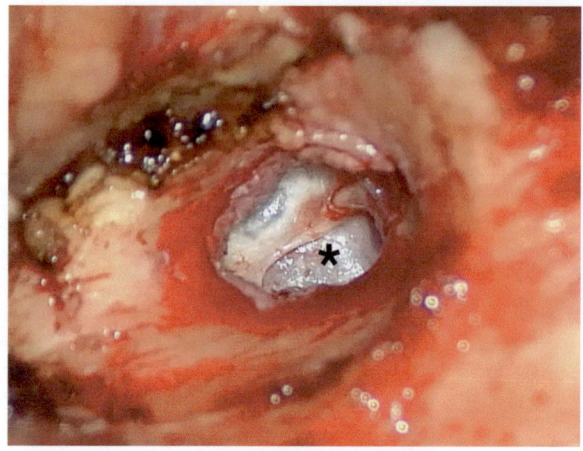

Fig. 11.12 At the beginning of the surgery, a retraction pocket (black asterisk) is clearly visualized. The patient complied also of a draining ear and a facial nerve weakness (grade III) ipsilaterally

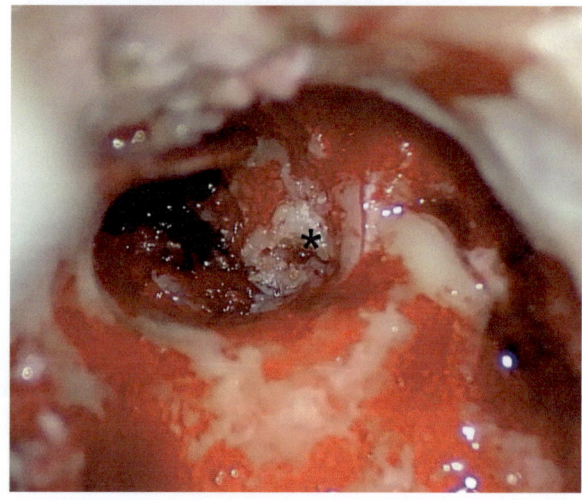

Fig. 11.13 Despite the complete anatomical control provided by the SP, the OW cannot be visualized. A "supposed" RW (black asterisk) is identified in close proximity of the tympanic portion of the facial nerve

Fig. 11.14 Even if in an anomalous relationship with the tympanic portion of facial nerve (black asterisk), consequence of the bony fragment displacement, the cochlear lumen is finally identified (white arrow)

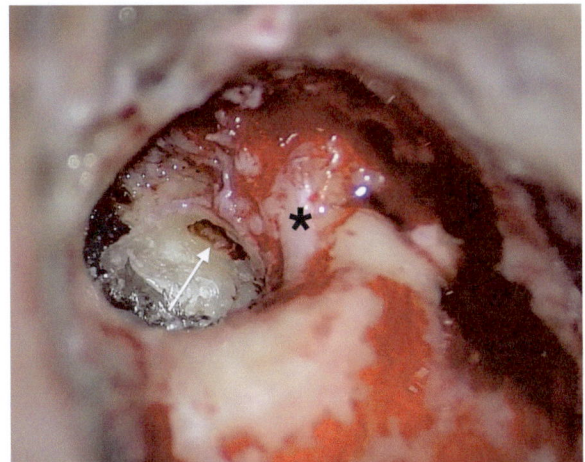

Fig. 11.15 After positioning of a depth-gauge, left temporarily in place to prevent blood and bone dust entering the cochlear lumen, the receiver-stimulator is positioned in its cradle

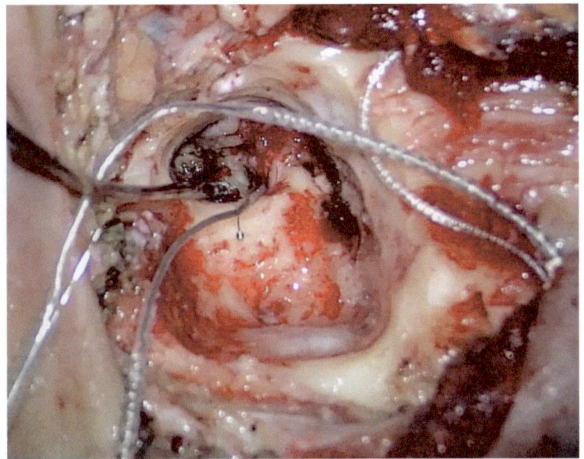

Fig. 11.16 Once the depth-gauge is removed, the array is immediately inserted in its final position

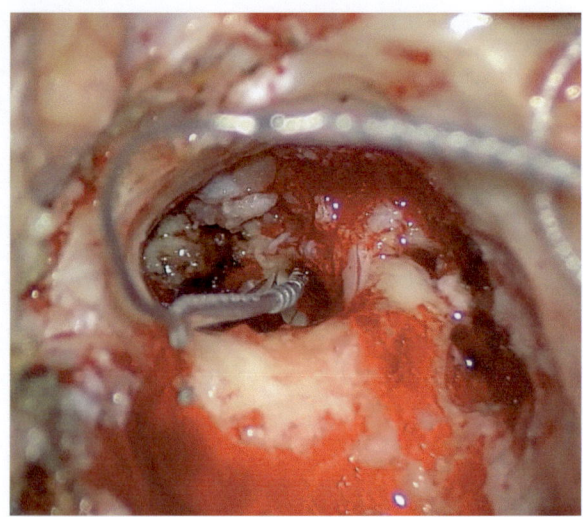

Fig. 11.17 Postoperative CT showing the correct positioning of the array

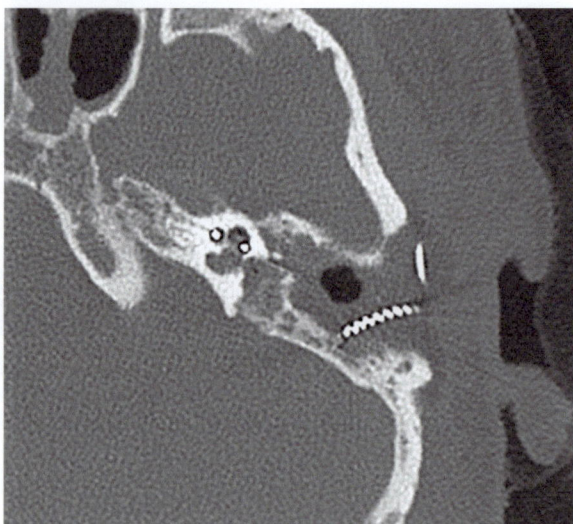

11 Temporal Bone Fractures and Otic Capsule Involvement: Surgical Tips in Cochlear... 129

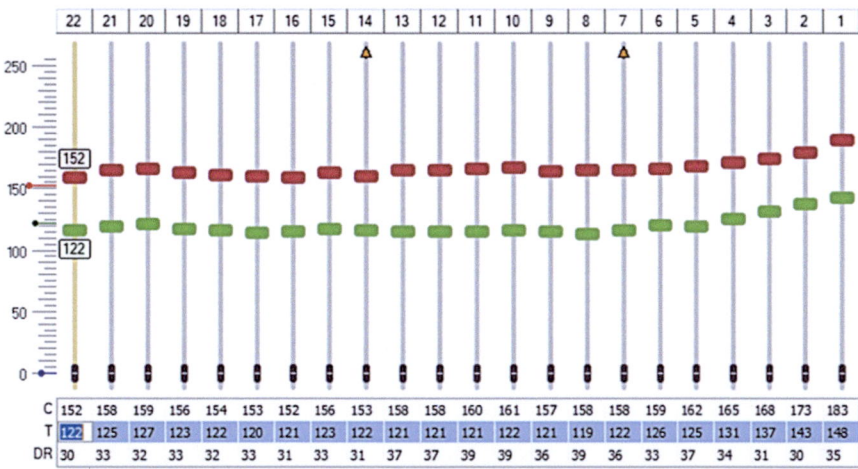

Fig. 11.18 In spite of the severe trauma with separation of the bony fragments, the residual ganglial cell population allows to reach sufficient level of stimulation

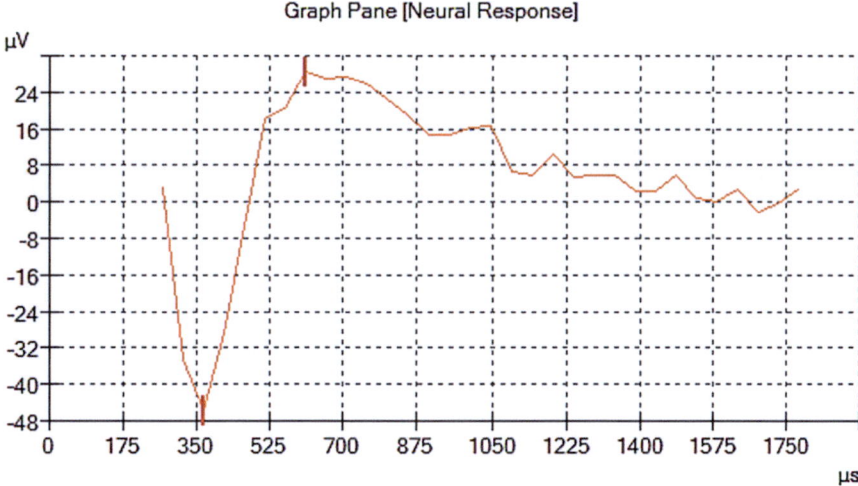

Fig. 11.19 The normal morphology and latency of the neural action potential, even if with a slight reduction of the amplitude, confirms a good depolarization of the fibers. Even in this case, the results were in agreement with the preoperative data recorded with the promontory test. The patient was able to reach good percentages of word and sentences recognition in open-set

References

1. Brodie HA, Thompson TC. Management of complications from 820 temporal bone fractures. PubMed. 1997;18(2):188–97.
2. Ishman SL, Friedland DR. Temporal bone fractures: traditional classification and clinical relevance. Laryngoscope. 2004;114(10):1734–41.
3. Sudhoff H, Linthicum FH. Temporal bone fracture and latent meningitis: temporal bone histopathology study of the month. Otol Neurotol. 2003;24(3):521–2.
4. Johnson F, Semaan MT, Megerian CA. Temporal bone fracture: evaluation and management in the modern era. Otolaryngol Clin North Am. 2008 Jun;41(3):597–618.
5. Sanna M. Surgery for cochlear and other auditory implants, 2015. Stuttgart: Thieme; 2015.
6. D'Angelo G, et al. Subtotal petrosectomy and cochlear implantation. Acta Otorhinolaryngologica Italica. 2020;40(6):450–6. https://doi.org/10.14639/0392-100x-n0931.

Vestibular Schwannomas and Intracoclear Schwannomas: Critical Factors in Cochlear Implantation

12

Cochlear implantation (CI) in vestibular schwannoma (VS) (Fig. 12.1)/neurofibromatotis type II (NF2) (Fig. 12.5) patients is a challenging procedure [1–4]. Multiple options are available: (1) implantation without tumor removal; (2) tumor removal with concomitant CI; (3) delayed CI after total/partial tumor removal and positioning of a depth gauge into the cochlea (Figs. 12.2, 12.3, and 12.4); (4) CI after a failed attempt of hearing preservation (even in this case, a promontorial test is strongly recommended). The decision-making is usually the most demanding task, as well as timing of the surgery. However, from a surgical point of view, the procedure does not differ very much from the standard one. It can be performed in the same stage of the tumor removal as well as in a second stage. If this latter option is preferred, positioning of a depth gauge in the cochlea during the first stage is suggested to avoid a complete cochlear ossification, a common occurrence in case of traumatization of the inner ear vascularization during tumor removal. In case of staged procedure, following a translabyrinthine approach, the second stage should be limited to the mastoid, avoiding reopening of the already sealed intradural space.

Because NF2 patients are routinely scheduled for radiological follow-up through magnetic resonance imaging (MRI), as in cases of cholesteatoma, the receiver-stimulator must be located in a more postero-superior position to reduce the shadow effect on the cerebello-pontine angle [5–7].

Of course, the surgery has only a minimal influence on the performances of the patients, with the amount of remaining functional nerve fibers being the most important factor.

Case 12.1 *Patient with diagnosis of right sided small vestibular schwannoma and poor preoperative hearing. After a few years of "wait and scan," due to the tumor growth, a translabyrinthine removal was scheduled, with attempt of cochlear nerve preservation.*

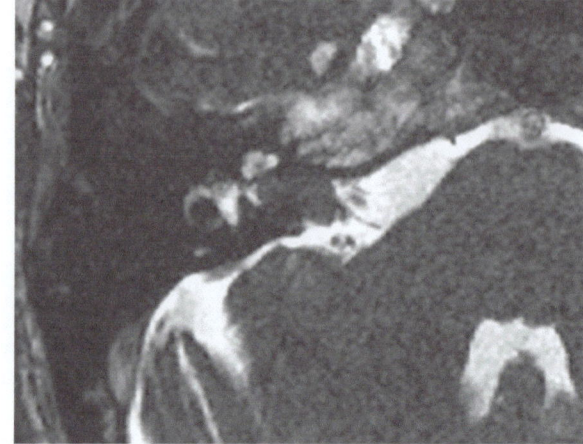

Fig. 12.1 RM showing a small vestibular schwannoma confined to the IAC

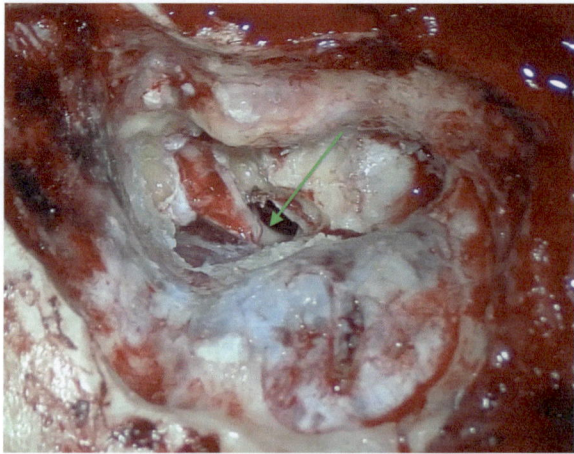

Fig. 12.2 Intraoperative view of the surgical field after the tumor removal, with the anatomical integrity of the cochlear nerve (green arrow)

Fig. 12.3 A posterior tympanotomy was drilled, the RW membrane identified and opened, and a depth gauge was left into the cochlea to preserve its lumen

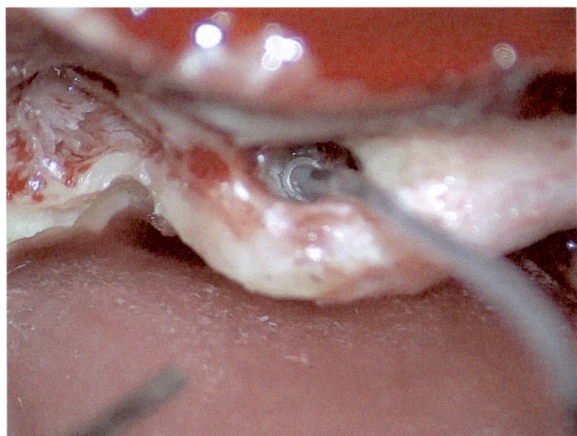

Fig. 12.4 A postoperative CT showed the amount of bone removal of the translabyrinthine approach as well as the correct position of the depth gauge. The promontory test performed 2 months after the surgery did not elicit any acoustic sensation and the second stage was then not performed

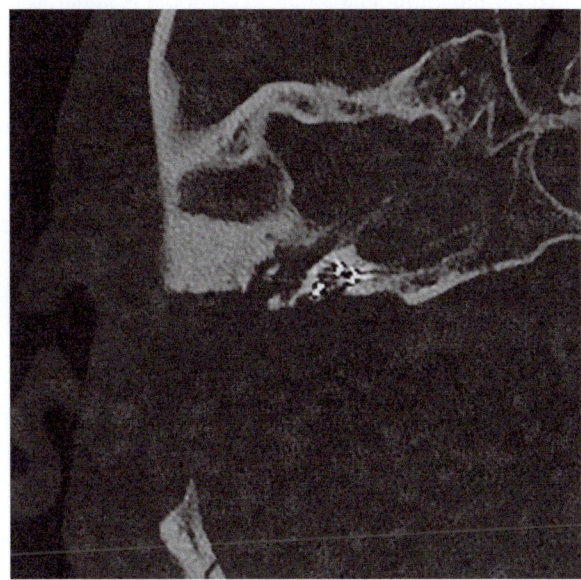

12.1 Intracochlear Schwannomas

Intracochlear schwannomas represent around 50% of all the intralabyrinthine schwannomas and may be found in the contest of a NF2 (Figs. 12.5, 12.6, 12.7, 12.8, 12.9, 12.10, and 12.11) or as isolated lesions (Figs. 12.12, 12.13, 12.14, 12.15, 12.16, 12.17, 12.18, 12.19, 12.20, 12.21, 12.22, and 12.23). Even in this case, the surgeon has the option to insert the CI with or without tumor removal [2]. The latter option may be achieved through the standard transmastoid approach, while the former requires a subtotal petrosectomy (SP) with a promontorium drill-out. The amount of drilling is indicated by the tumor consistency (some lesions may be just pulled out en-block, others are very fragile and necessitate a peace-meal removal) and the extension of the lesion into the cochlear turns. In case of complete cochlea involvement by a fragile tumor, to avoid a total drill-out, after exposure of the basal turn, the surgeon may create a small opening at the level of the middle turn. A depth gauge introduced into the basal turn is then progressively pushed superiorly into the cochlear lumen in an attempt to drive the residual tumor to the second opening in the middle turn, where it can be removed (Fig. 12.8) [3]. A staged procedure has been described even in this case, always leaving a depth gauge into the cochlear lumen [4]. The authors prefer to select this latter option only in case where the patient is not convinced of the application of the CI, only to keep an open door for the future.

In cases of cochlear implantation in intracochlear vestibular schwannomas, in order to foresee the performance level from the cochlear implant, it is mandatory to perform a correct preoperative evaluation of the cochlear nerve function.

Promontory testing should be used in the presurgical phase, determining a range of stimulation and the related responses over a wide frequency range (from 50 to 1600 Hz). Furthermore, the electrophysiological evaluation may also differentiate between lesions sparing the nerve ganglion fibers and those involving them. This represents one of the most important parameters, together with the intracochlear extension of the tumor and the surgical damage necessary for its removal, that influences the result of the cochlear implantation in this patients.

Case 12.2 NF2 patient with bilateral tumors and an additional intracochlear lesion on the left side. Before planning a removal of the large tumor on the right (the only hearing ear), a CI was positioned on the left side, leaving in place the cerebellopontine angle lesion and removing only the intracochlear tumor.

12.1 Intracochlear Schwannomas

Fig. 12.5 RM, high-resolution T2 sequences, showing an area of absence of intracochlear fluid at the level of the basal turn of the scala tympani (white arrow) on the left side (compare with the contralateral side)

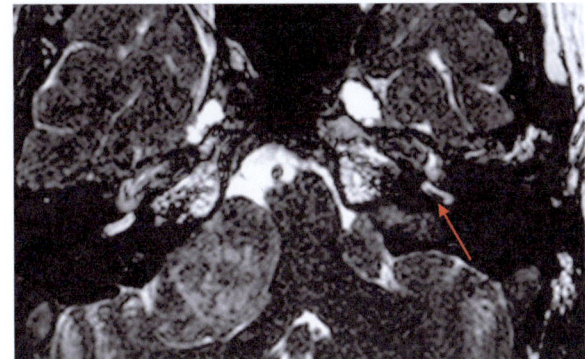

Fig. 12.6 An SP has been completed, the cochlear lumen opened, and the tumor in the basal turn visualized (white arrow). Due to its consistency, being hooked and pulled posteriorly, it came out without fragmentation

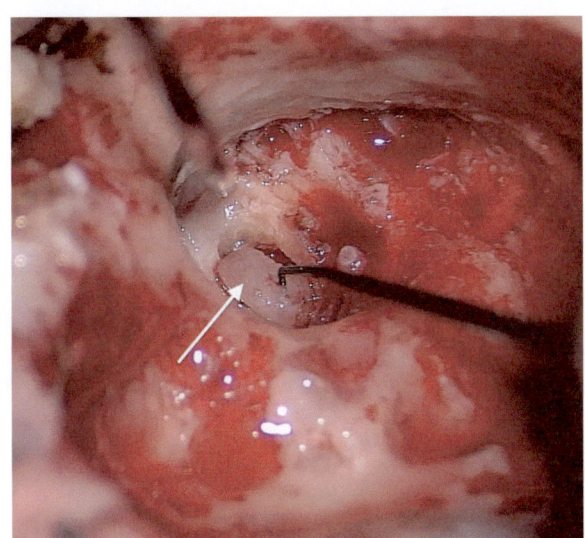

Fig. 12.7 After tumor removal, both the scala tympani and the scala vestibuli are clearly visible. The basial membrane and the lamina cribrosa at the level of the lesion are not visible anymore

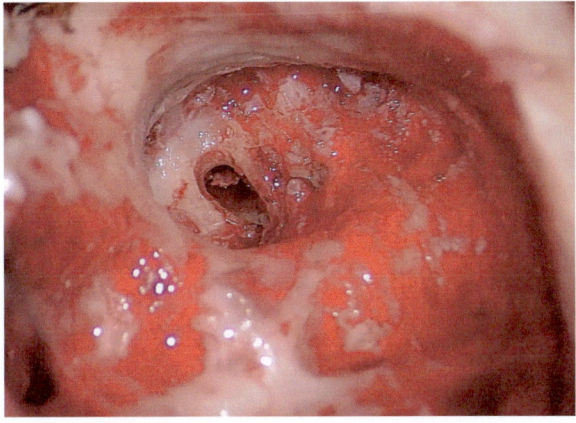

Fig. 12.8 A complete array insertion has been finally accomplished

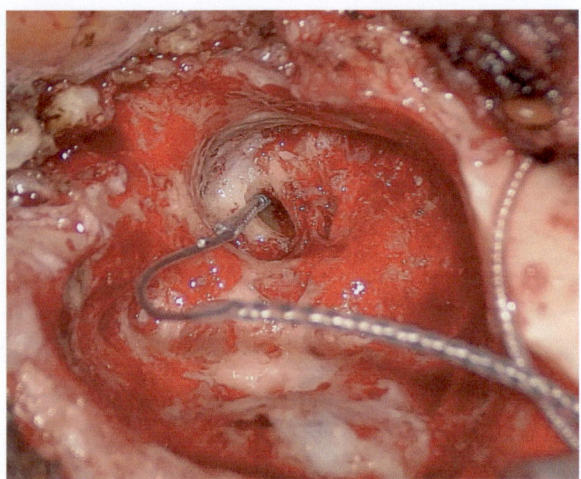

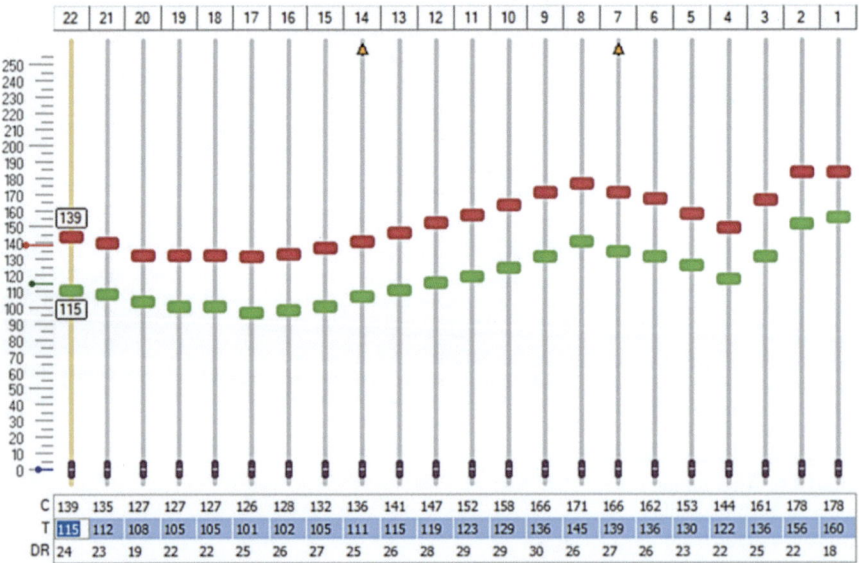

Fig. 12.9 Stimulation levels are higher in the basal turn of the cochlea (directly involved by the tumor and the surgical trauma). Nonetheless, open-set speech recognition at 6 months follow-up reaches 90% at 65 dB SPL in silence

12.1 Intracochlear Schwannomas

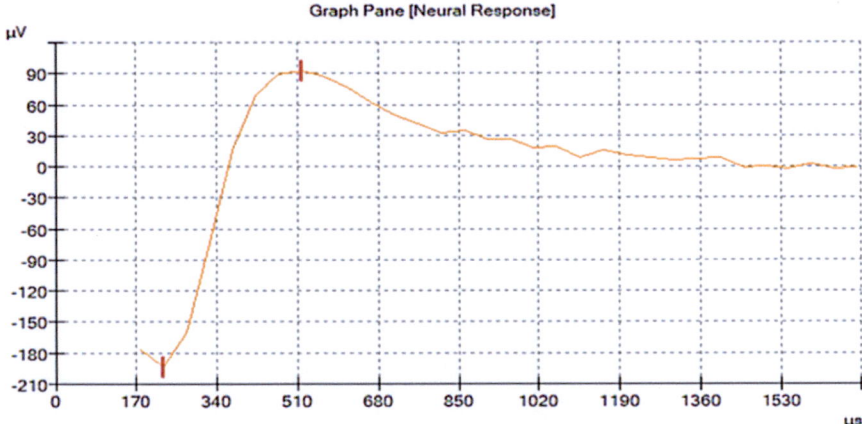

Fig. 12.10 The neural action potential was detected over all the electrodes. However, better responses could be observed at middle and apical turn level (picture showing electrode 16)

Fig. 12.11 The EABR shows a preserved synchronization of the nerve fibers depolarization, even if the cerebellopontine angle tumor is still in place

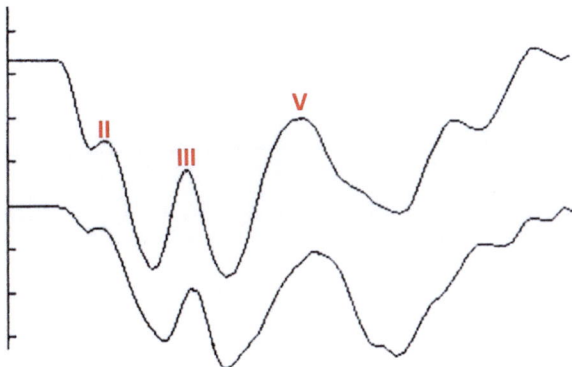

Case 3 *Patient affected by an intracochlear schwannoma filling the majority of the cochlea. The lesion was removed through an SP combined with a labyrinthectomy. It was possible to partially preserve the bony cochlear anatomy and a CI was then positioned.*

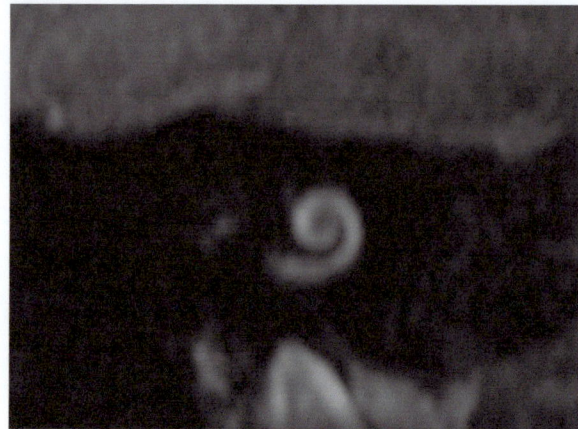

Fig. 12.12 MRI showing an intracochlear schwannoma with complete cochlear invasion

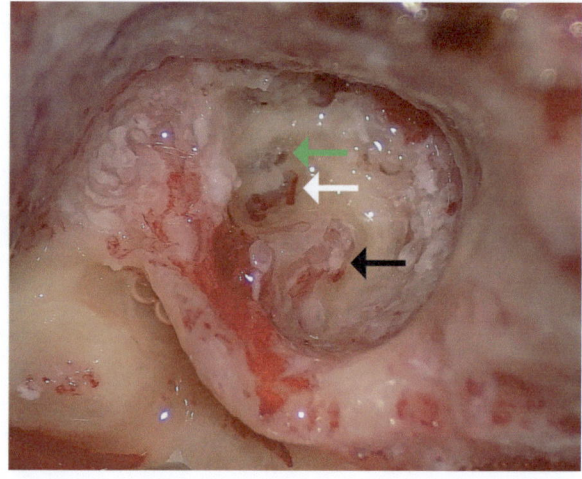

Fig. 12.13 A labyrinthectomy has been combined with the standard SP. Drilling of the promontorium allowed identification of all the three cochlear turns. Basal turn (black arrow), middle turn (white arrow), apical turn (green arrow)

12.1 Intracochlear Schwannomas

Fig. 12.14 After opening of the lateral aspect of the basal turn, the tumor (black asterisk) is visualized

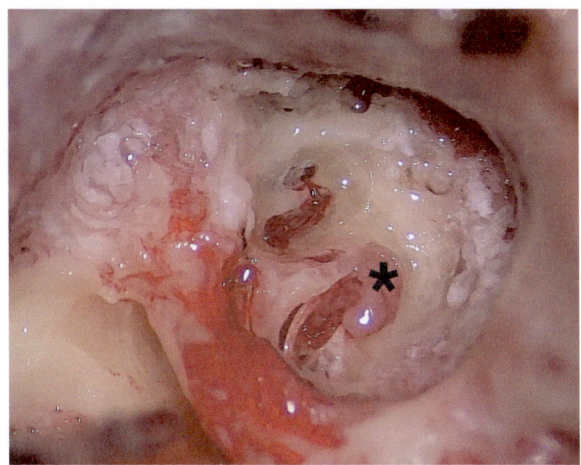

Fig. 12.15 The tumor (black asterisk) removal starts at the level of the basal turn

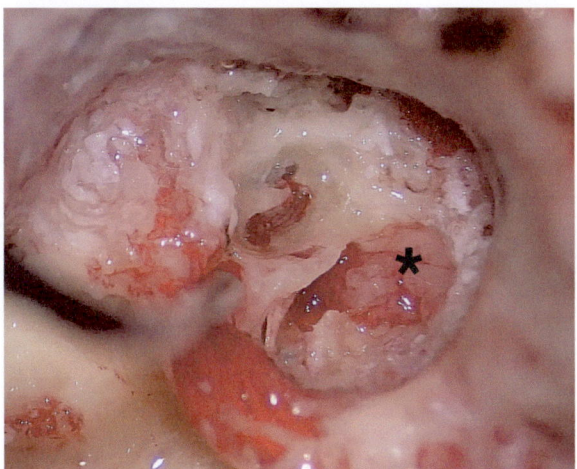

Fig. 12.16 The tumor (black asterisk) is then removed from the middle and apical turn

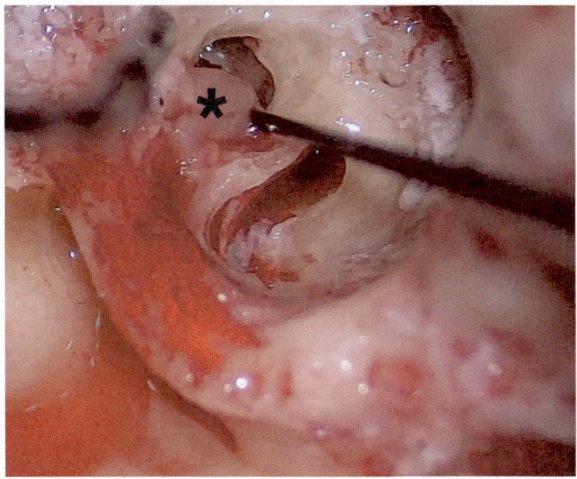

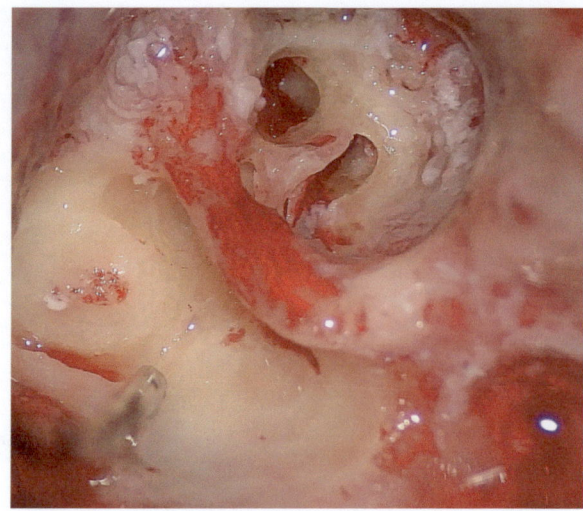

Fig. 12.17 The aspect of the open cochlea after the tumor removal. Note that the tumor mass and surgical maneuvers have partially destroyed the interscalar septum between the middle and the apical turn

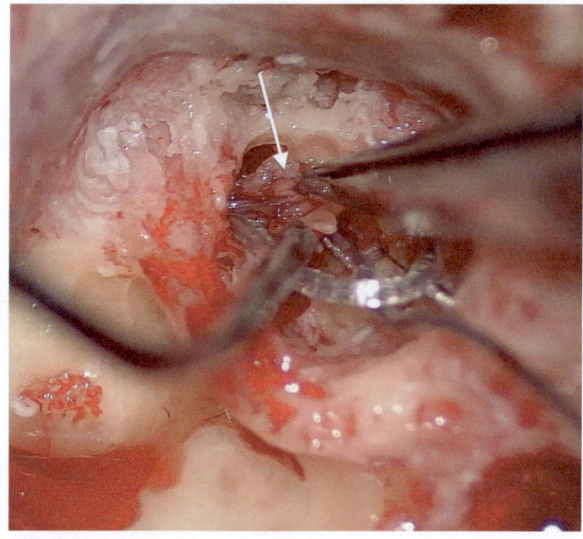

Fig. 12.18 A depth gauge is inserted into the cochlear lumen and pushed till the apical turn. The maneuver drives some small tumor remnants (white arrow) left into the medial aspect of the cochlea until reaching the opening created at the level of the middle turn. Once there, they are easily removed

12.1 Intracochlear Schwannomas

Fig. 12.19 Before final array insertion, the cochlea is inspected with the help of an endoscope, confirming the preservation of the inner anatomy

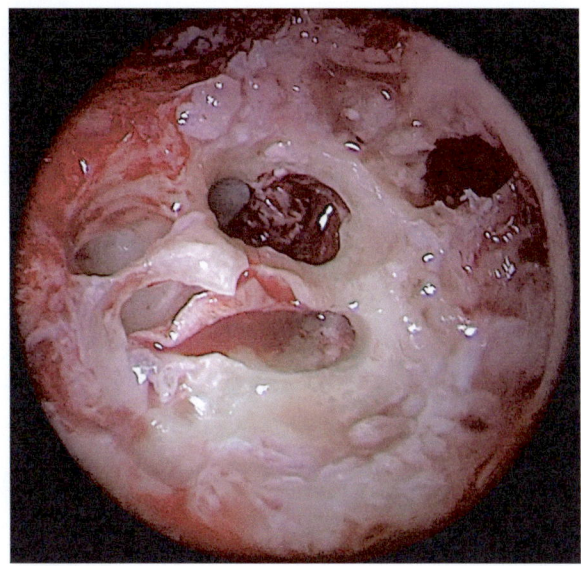

Fig. 12.20 All the array electrodes have been positioned into the cochlear lumen

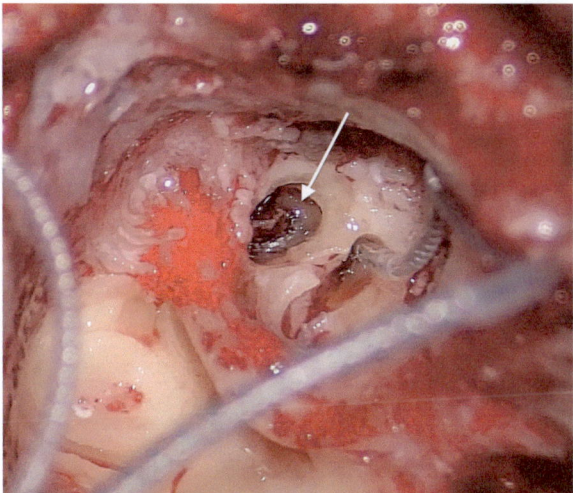

Fig. 12.21 Postoperative CT confirming the correct array insertion. Note the electrodes into the middle turn of the cochlea (white arrow)

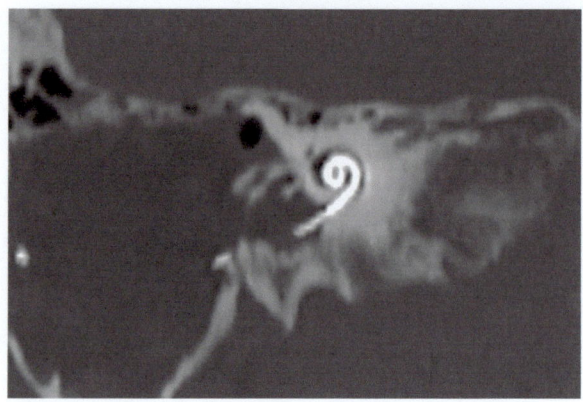

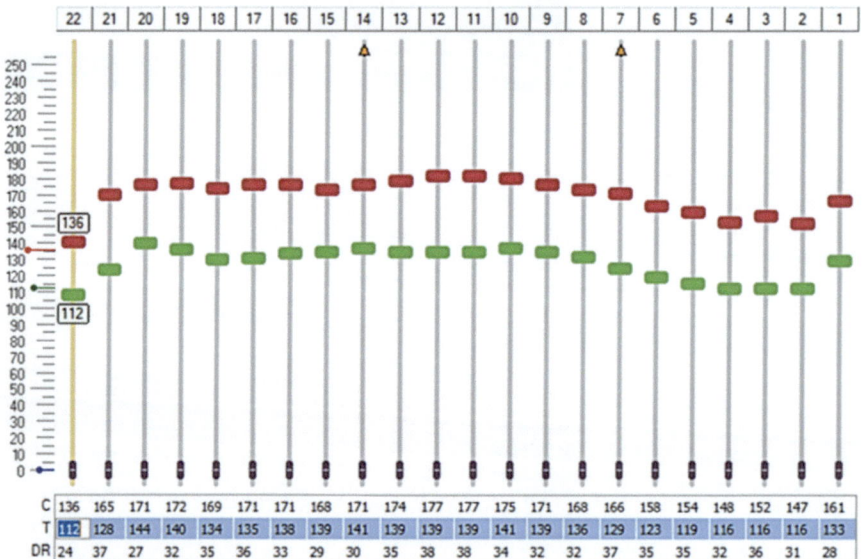

Fig. 12.22 In spite of the aggressive surgery, the stimulation levels are comparable to those obtained after a standard cochlear implantation procedure in a normal cochlea

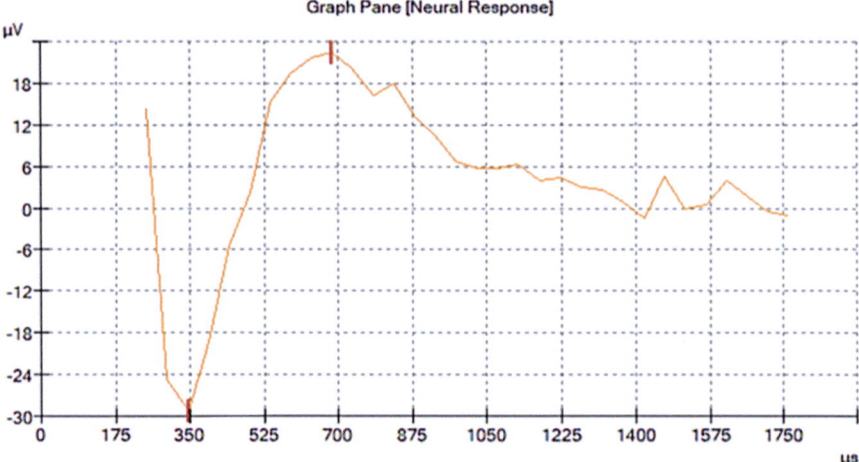

Fig. 12.23 Nerve action potential was detected over all the cochlear implant electrodes, showing the lack of involvement of the nerve ganglion. Open-set speech recognition reached 100% at 65 dB SPL

References

1. Grenier B, Mosnier I, Ferrary E, Nguyen Y, Sterkers O, Kalamarides M, et al. Cochlear implantation in neurofibromatosis type 2-related schwannomatosis: long-term hearing outcomes. Otolaryngology. 2024;171(1):218–30.
2. Carlson ML, Breen JT, Colin LMJ, Neff BA, Gifford RH, et al. Cochlear implantation in patients with neurofibromatosis type 2. 2012;33(5):853–62.
3. Lustig LR, Yeagle J, Driscoll CLW, Blevins N, Francis H, Niparko JK. Cochlear implantation in patients with neurofibromatosis type 2 and bilateral vestibular schwannoma. Otol Neurotol. 2006;27(4):512–8.
4. Carlson ML, Neff BA, Sladen DP, Link MJ, Driscoll CL. Cochlear implantation in patients with intracochlear and intralabyrinthine schwannomas. Otol Neurotol. 2016;37(6):647–53.
5. Liaci E, Bertoli G, Lella FD, Falcioni M. Intralabyrinthine schwannoma: surgical management and cochlear lumen preservation. Am J Otolaryngol. 2023;45(2):104158.
6. Iannaccone FP, Rahne T, Zanoletti E, Plontke SK. Cochlear implantation in patients with inner ear schwannomas: a systematic reviewed meta-analysis of audiological outcomes. Our Arch Otorhinolaryngol. 2024;281(12):6175–86.
7. Davis NL, Rappaport JM, MacDougall JC. Cochlear and auditory brainstem implants in the management of acoustic neuroma and bilateral acoustic neurofibromatosis. McGill J Med. 2020;3(2)

Cochlear Implant Positioning in Atypical Otological Scenarios

13

A cochlear implant may be indicated in a lot of rare and "anomalous" situations; in this case, the decision should take into consideration the real necessity of the implant for audiological reasons, the difficulties in reopening the surgical cavity if the implant becomes necessary in the future (for example in presence of a graft for facial nerve reconstruction like in case 13.1), and the obstacle represented by the implant when a postoperative FU requires the patient to undergo an MRI [1].

The combination of a labyrinthectomy with a CI procedure, usually adopted in Meniere disease with profound sensorineural hearing loss and persisting vertigo spells, can be performed through the classic transmastoid approach [2, 3]. However, if required from additional problems, a labyrinthectomy (Figs. 13.16, 13.17, 13.18, 13.19, 13.20, 13.21, 13.22, 13.23) or even a translabyrinthine approach (Figs. 13.1, 13.2, 13.3, 13.4, 13.5, 13.6, 13.7, 13.8, and 13.9) can also be easily combined with the SP and a cochlear implantation without any difficulties.

In a rare case of a CI implanted after a brainstem implant, the main difficulties are not represented by the surgery, but by cortical area rearrangement with a new tonotopicity artificially created through the ABI stimulation [4]. With the CI, a second rearrangement must be obtained, because of another change in the neural activity due to the different synchronicity of depolarization of the cochlear nerve fibers. The patients need to readapt to a new and more precise acoustic message, and this process may take a long time [5]. This process is simpler and faster if the ABI did not work properly (see case 11.1 in Chap. 11). The only surgical problem may be represented by the necessity to find a room for an additional receiver-stimulator in case the ABI should be maintained in place (Figs. 13.10, 13.11, 13.12, 13.13, 13.14, and 13.15).

Case 13.1 *Petrous bone cholestetoma with preoperative facial palsy in a patient already treated with a canal wall-down tympanoplasty. In such a situation, the CI should be considered an option in young patients, when a facial nerve graft is positioned in the cavity and the majority of the cochlea is still spared by the lesion, without necessity to be drilled away for radicality. The advantages of the hearing rehabilitation must be balanced with the impossibility to use the diffusion-weighted MRI sequences in the follow-up.*

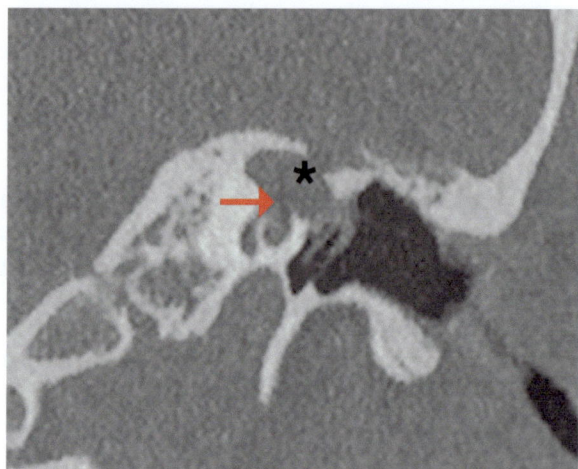

Fig. 13.1 Coronal CT scan showing a supralabyrinthine cholesteatoma (black asterisk) with minimal cochlea erosion (green arrow). The patient already had undergone a canal wall-down technique

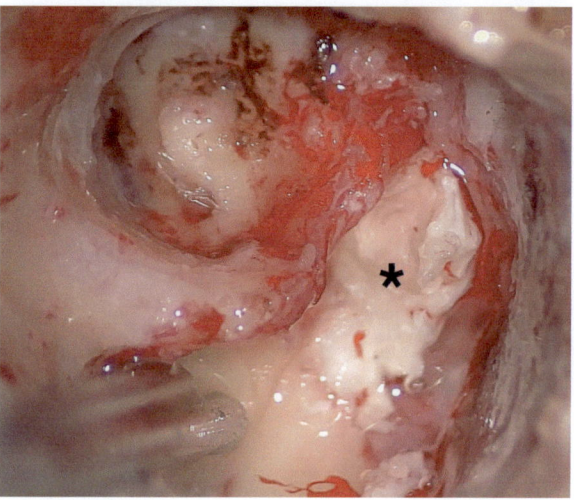

Fig. 13.2 Intraoperative, the cholesteatoma (black asterisk) is exposed through an SP combined with a labyrintectomy

Fig. 13.3 After cholesteatoma removal, the facial nerve is reconstructed by means of a great auricular nerve graft (black asterisks)

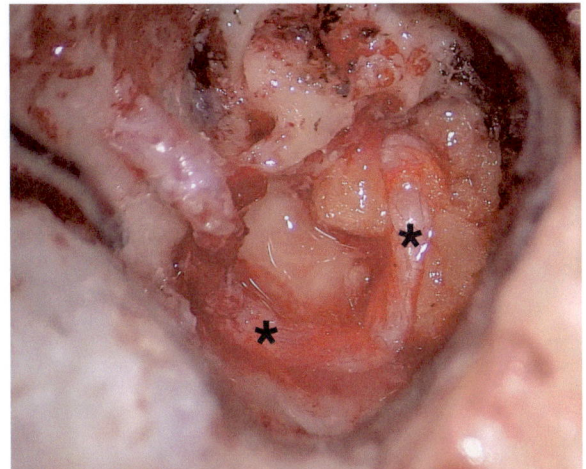

Fig. 13.4 The nerve graft is protected with some abdominal fat (black asterisk) and the RW opened (white arrow)

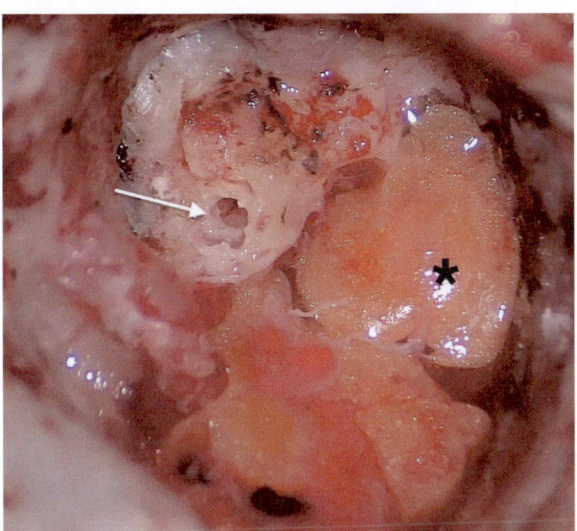

Fig. 13.5 The array is fully inserted without difficulties. Additional fat will be interposed in between the graft and the connecting cable

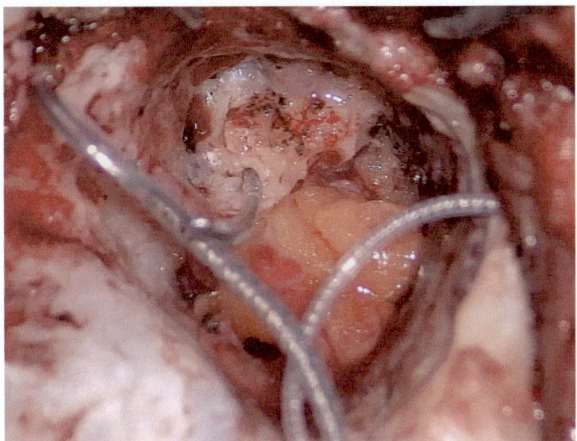

Fig. 13.6 Postoperative CT reconstructed along the cochlear planes. In spite of the partial erosion of the cochlea, the array is correctly positioned

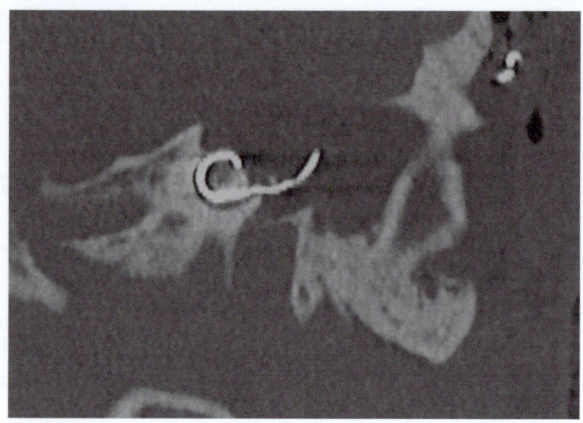

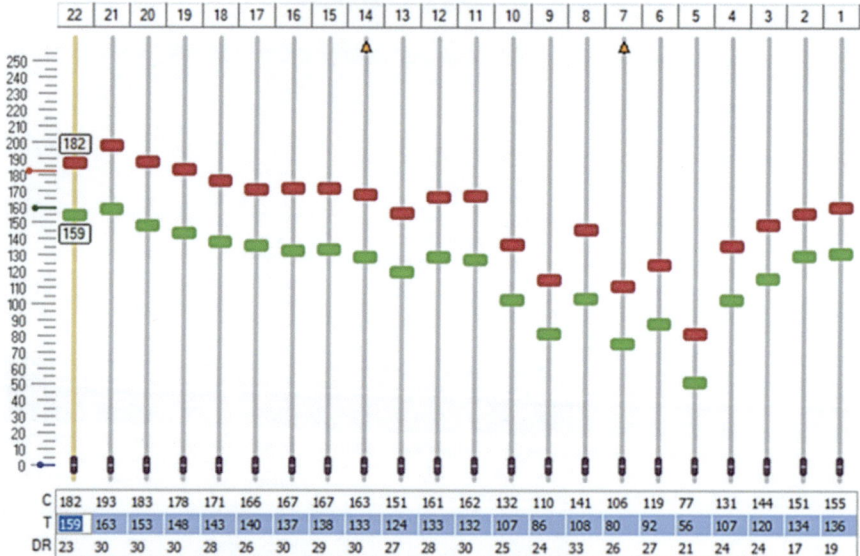

Fig. 13.7 Even if all the electrodes have been activated, the map shows a large variability of the stimulation levels. This feature may also been influenced by some surgical manipulation of the cochlear nerve occurred into the fundus of the internal auditory canal while preparing the central stump of the facial nerve for grafting, or by the partial cochlear erosion

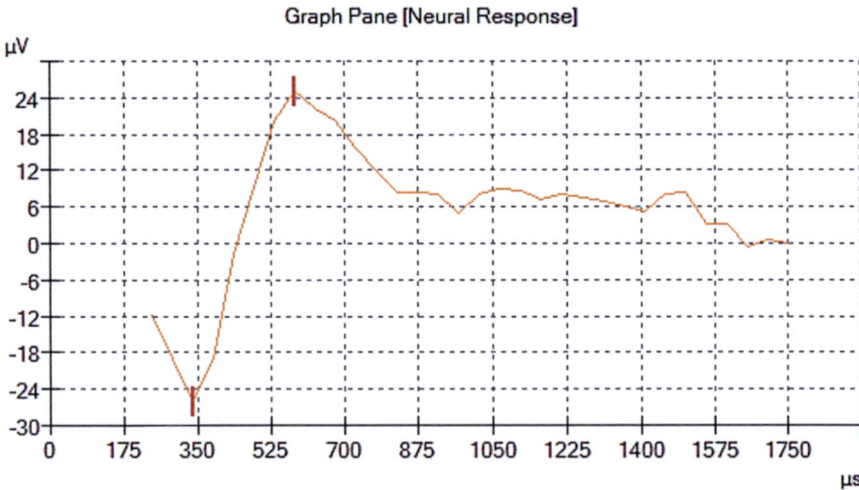

Fig. 13.8 In agreement with the map on Fig. 13.7, it was possible to elicit a very good action nerve potential from the electrodes 1–14, positioned at the basal and middle cochlear turn

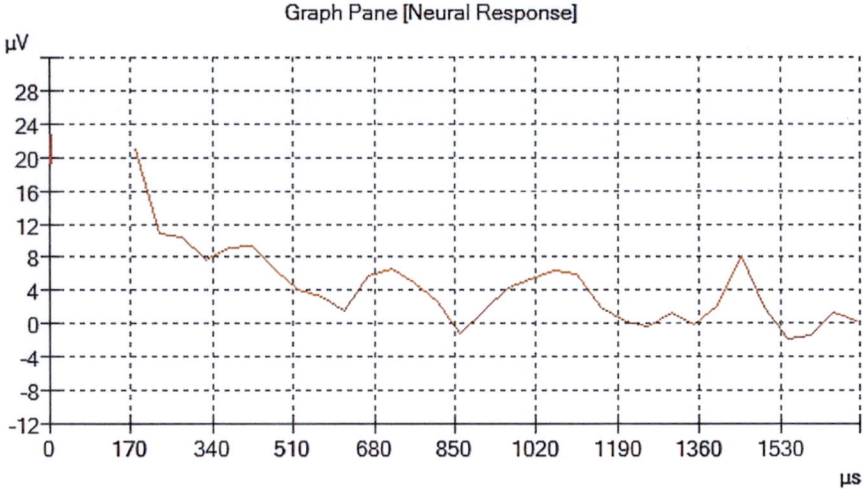

Fig. 13.9 The neural potential did not have the same good parameters or was not clearly detected on electrodes 15–22

Case 13.2 *CI following an ipsilateral ABI. The reason for implanting the brainstem instead of the cochlea by the previous surgeon was not clear. The ABI had 16 active electrodes, initially, and the patient could reach 60% of word discrimination in open set. However, with time, the performances progressively decreased till simple sound detection that the patient did not want to lose. The surgical procedure did not show any particular difficulty, but the necessity to maintain in place the ABI, in order to let it work in case of unsuccessful cochlear implantation.*

However, for the aforementioned difficulties, it took almost 24 months for the patient to reach the standard word and speech recognition performances.

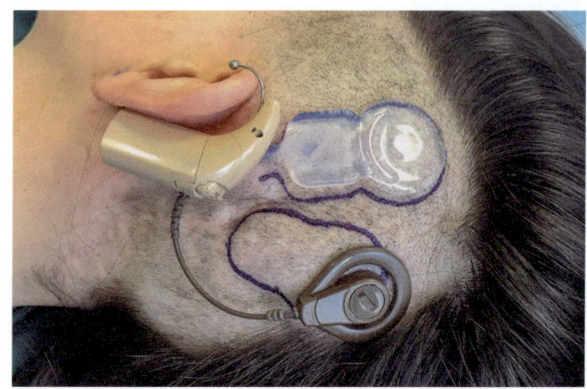

Fig. 13.10 The position of the old (posterior) and the new receiver-stimulator (anterior) is outlined on the skin before surgery

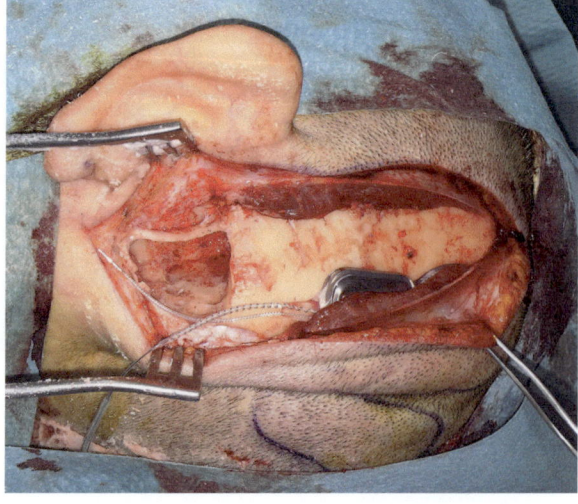

Fig. 13.11 The skin incision runs more anteriorly to accommodate the new receiver-stimulator without the need to remove the old one. The mastoidectomy has been completed and the receiver-stimulator positioned in place

13 Cochlear Implant Positioning in Atypical Otological Scenarios

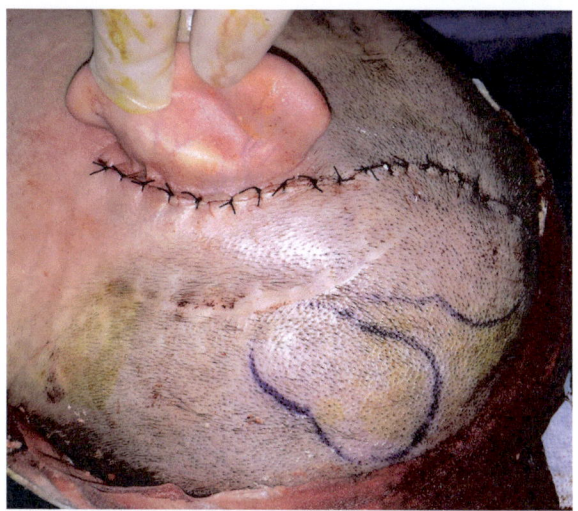

Fig. 13.12 The operation is completed without disturbing the receiver-stimulator of the brainstem implant

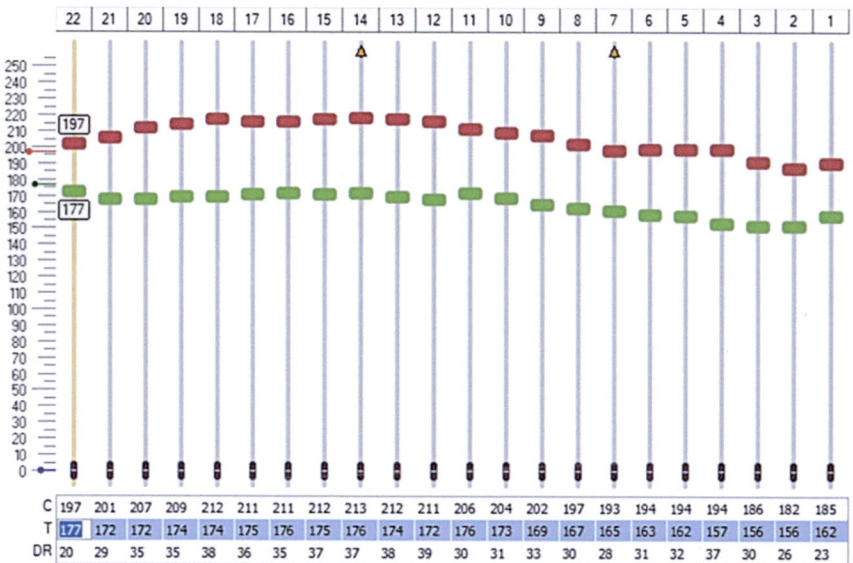

Fig. 13.13 The high levels of stimulation showed on the map are difficult to be explained; probably they are influenced by the previous prolonged use of a brainstem implant (around 14 years). Even if after a long delay (2 years), the patient was able to reach very good performances in word and sentences recognition in open set

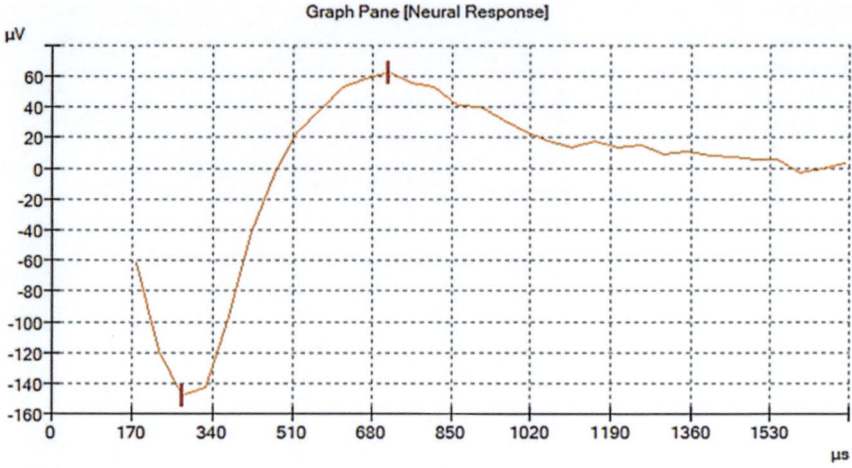

Fig. 13.14 The nerve action potential confirms a good fiber depolarization on all the electrodes

Fig. 13.15 The graphic shows an EABR with morphology, waves amplitude, and latencies in the normal range, confirming a good neural conductivity

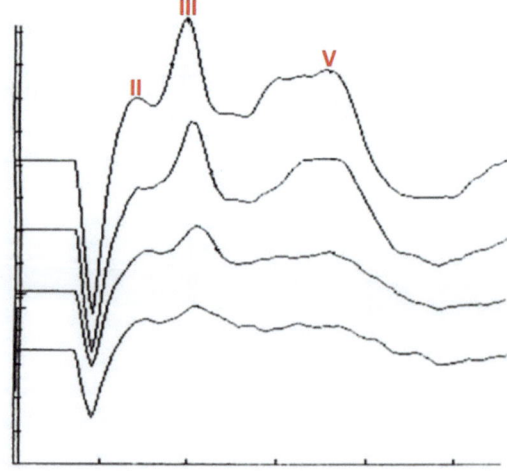

13 Cochlear Implant Positioning in Atypical Otological Scenarios

Case 13.3 *Fracture of the otic capsule with dead ear, post-traumatic cholesteatoma, and delayed vertigo. An SP combined with a labyrinthectomy was planned to manage all the problems in the same stage. The surgery was also made more complex by the presence of a basal turn ossification.*

Fig. 13.16 Axial CT scan showing a fracture line (white arrow) crossing the left vestibule. Some soft tissue (black arrow) is also detected antero-medial to the head of the malleus

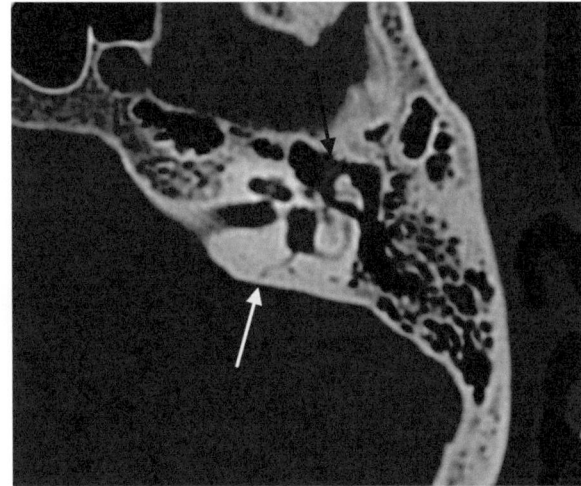

Fig. 13.17 3D MRI reconstruction confirms the presence of labyrinthine fluids into the cochlea (white arrow). On the contrary, the semicircular canals are completely obliterated

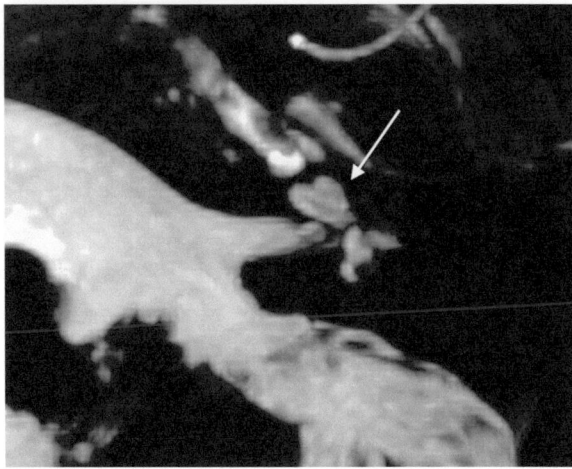

Fig. 13.18 Otoscopic view of the left ear showing both cholesteatoma and tympanosclerosis

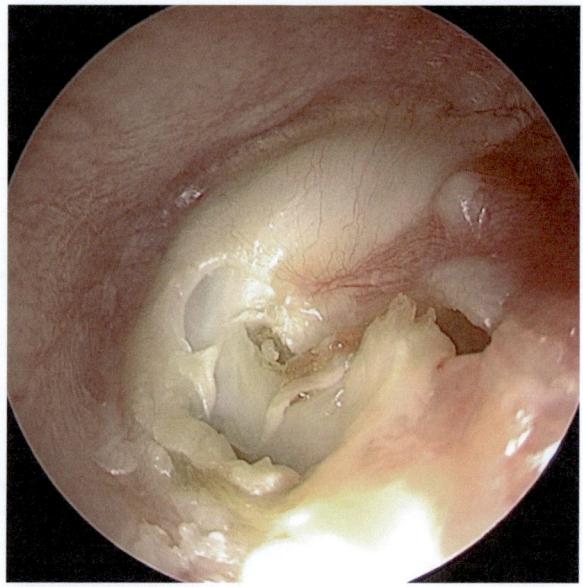

Fig. 13.19 Intraoperatively some cholesteatoma is detected and removed medial to the malleus head (black asterisk)

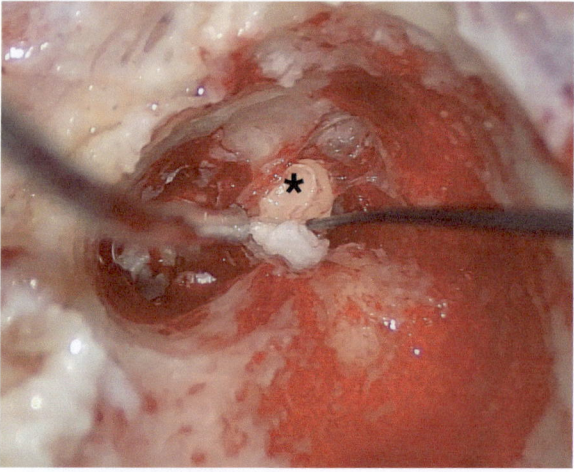

Fig. 13.20 As detected by the MRI images, the semicircular canals are completely obliterated by fibrotic tissue partially ossified. Superior semicircular canal (black arrow), lateral semicircular canal (white arrow)

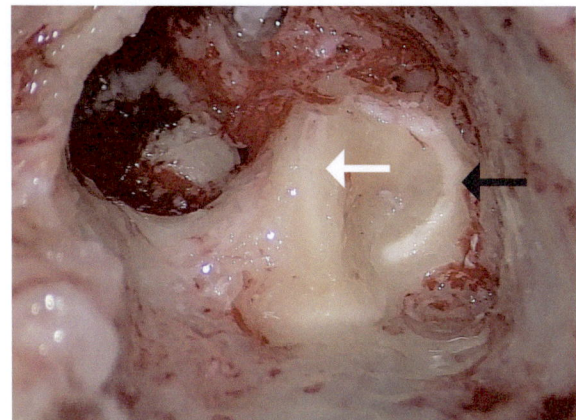

Fig. 13.21 The SP and the labyrinthectomy have been accomplished. The RW is opened. Medial wall of the vestibule (black asterisk), facial nerve (white asterisk)

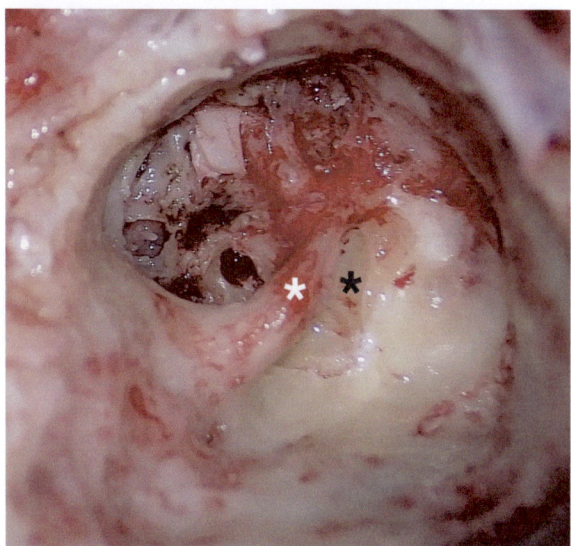

Fig. 13.22 A full array insertion is accomplished

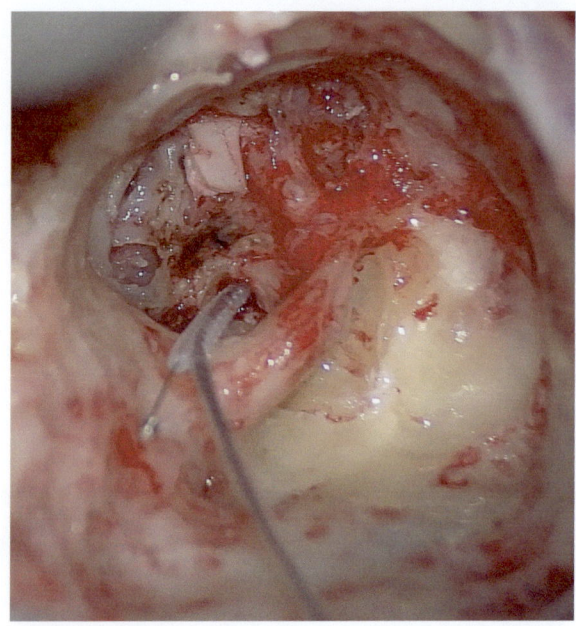

Fig. 13.23 Postoperative CT scan confirming the correct array placement. Note the drilling of the vestibule (white asterisk)

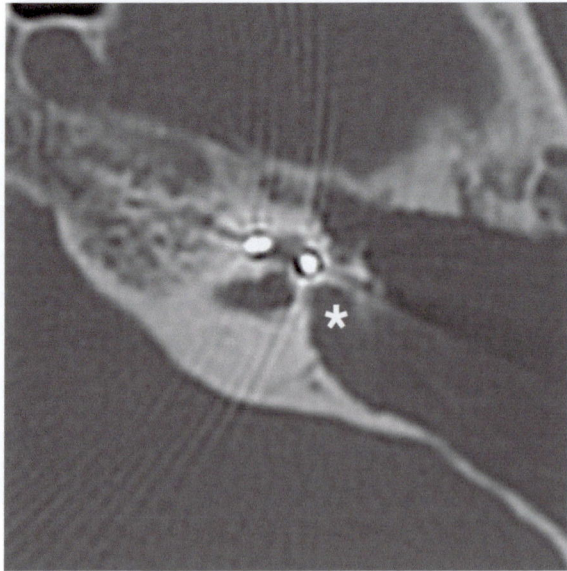

References

1. Lassig AAD, Zwolan TA, Telian SA. Cochlear implant failures and revision. Otol Neurotol. 2005;26(4):624–34.
2. Zwolan TA, Shepard NT, Niparko JK. Labyrinthectomy with cochlear implantation. PubMed. 1993;14(3):220–3.
3. Perkins E, Rooth M, Dillon M, Brown K. Simultaneous labyrinthectomy and cochlear implantation in unilateral meniere's disease. Laryngoscope Invest Otolaryngol. 2018;3(3):225–30.
4. Vincenti V, Pasanisi E, Guida M, Di Trapani G, Sanna M. Hearing rehabilitation in neurofibromatosis type 2 patients: cochlear versus auditory brainstem implantation. Audiol Neurotol. 2008;13(4):273–80.
5. Merkus P, Lella FD, Trapani GD, Pasanisi E, Beltrame MA, Zanetti D, et al. Indications and contraindications of auditory brainstem implants: systematic review and illustrative cases. Eur Arch Oto Rhino Laryngol [Internet]. 2014;271(1):3–13.

Long-Term Follow-Up and Complication Management After Cochlear Implantation in Complex Otologic Cases

14.1 Follow-Up

Standard follow-up for CI patients usually includes otoscopy, electrophysiology, audiology, and logopedic evaluation. However, many difficult cases, especially when treated through an SP, require also a periodic radiological evaluation through a computed tomography scan (CT) or magnetic resonance imaging (MRI) (or a combination) [1]. The choice between CT and MRI depends on different factors such as the approach, the original disease, and the age of the patient (it is advisable not to perform a CT scan in young patients if not absolutely necessary, due to the risk related to radiation-induced lesions) [2].

Here is presented the author's follow-up protocol for those cases treated through an SP:

1. Children <12 years: no radiological investigations are routinely planned till they reach 12 years of age if not suspecting some complication.
2. Adults without preoperative skin in the surgical cavity: a CT scan is obtained in the immediate postoperative days to be used as a baseline for further control. In the absence of any audiological/otological issues, the patient undergoes another CT scan in between 5 and 7 years after the surgery. On the contrary, a CT scan is immediately repeated in presence of any anomalies or unexplained reduction of the performances.
3. Adult patients with preoperative skin (cholesteatoma or canal wall-down technique) in the surgical field: a CT scan is obtained in the immediate postoperative days to be used as a baseline for further control. A new CT scan is repeated every 3 years until 10 years from surgery to exclude the presence of iatrogenic cholesteatomas or cholesterol granulomas. Even if not specific for soft tissue, the CT scan may show suspect bony erosions not present at the baseline scan, as well as spheric areas of soft tissue with a different density if compared to the fat (Figs. 14.1 and 14.2).

Fig. 14.1 Postoperative CT-scan after a CI positioned in the contest of a SP plus labyrinthectomy

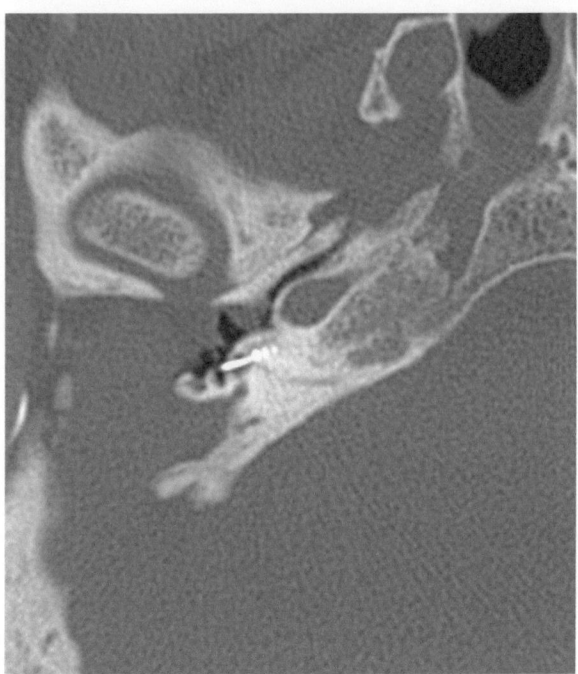

Fig. 14.2 Control CT-scan 5 years after the previous one (Fig. 14.1); note the bony erosion (white asterisk) occurred posteriorly to the mastoid portion of the facial nerve

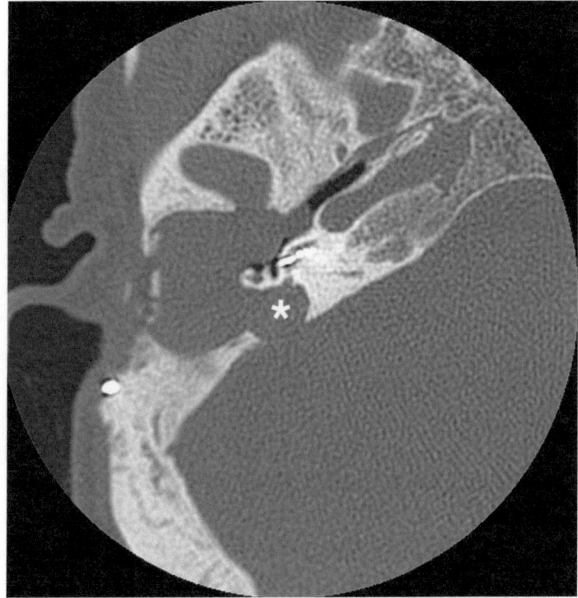

Fig. 14.3 MRI DWI sequences with a CI in place. The artifact obscures even the majority of the contralateral temporal bone

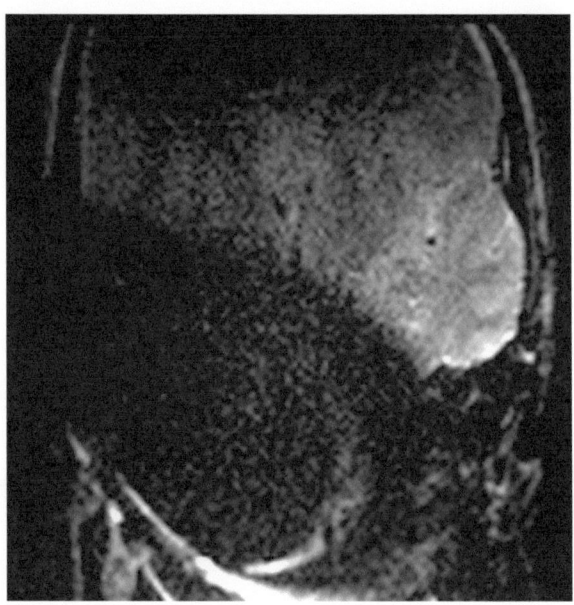

4. Adult patients with high risk of residual lesions (petrous bone cholesteatoma) in addition to the protocol at point 3: an MRI is planned after 6/7 years; in doubtful cases, the MR may be repeated after removal of the magnet (if possible) or the year after.

Even if nowadays the gold standard for detection of residual cholesteatoma is represented by the diffusion-weighted non-EPI MRI [3], the huge artifact produced by these sequences in presence of a CI makes the scan completely unreadable bilaterally (Fig. 14.3); for the ipsilateral temporal bone, this is true even after removal of the magnet (Fig. 14.4). Alternative sequences as T1 and T2, even if not specific for cholesteatoma, elicit less artifact and can be used (Figs. 14.5 and 14.6). For these sequences, the scans after magnet removal present only minimal/no artifacts. (Fig. 14.7). The need for an MRI, even if possible with the last generations of implants, must be balanced with a minimal risk of magnet dislocation (Fig. 14.8). Even magnet removal and repositioning must be reserved to cases with a high suspect of complications, in order to avoid unnecessary manipulation of the receiver-stimulator [4]. Multiple MR must be reserved only to particular cases.

Fig. 14.4 Same case of Fig. 14.3. MRI DWI sequences with a CI in place after magnet removal. The artifact is reduced but anyway obscures completely the ipsilateral temporal bone

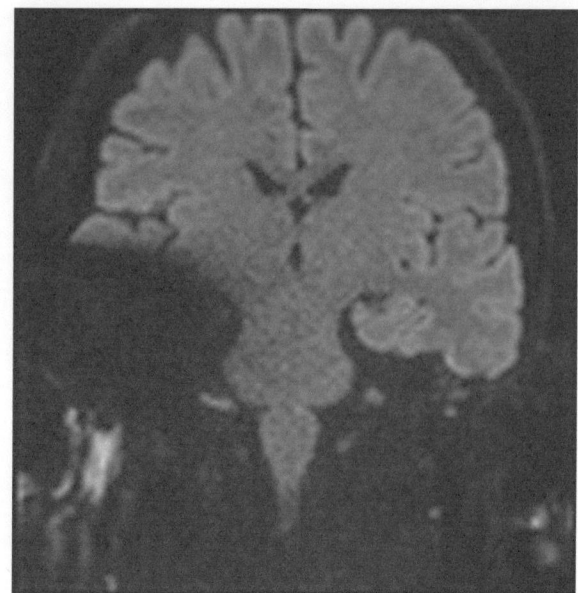

Fig. 14.5 Same case of Figs. 14.3 and 14.4. MRI T1 sequences with a CI in place. Even if with some distortion, the temporal bone is visible

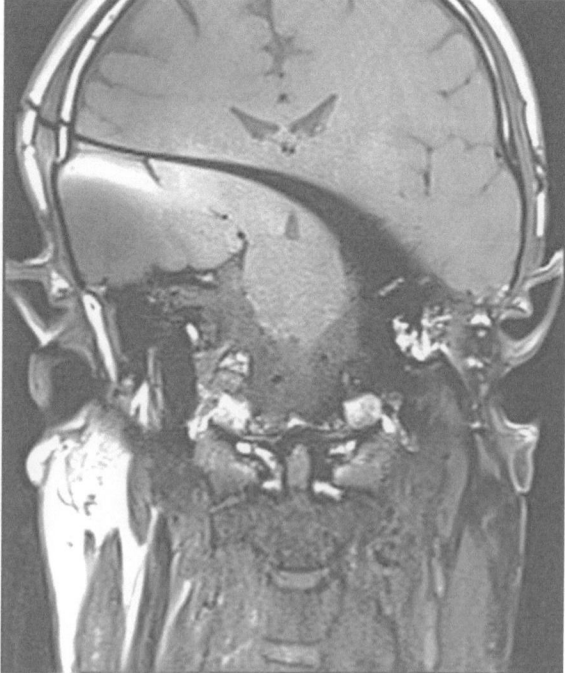

14.1 Follow-Up

Fig. 14.6 Same case of Figs. 14.3, 14.4, and 14.5. MRI T2 sequences with a CI in place. The temporal bone is visible with minimal distortion

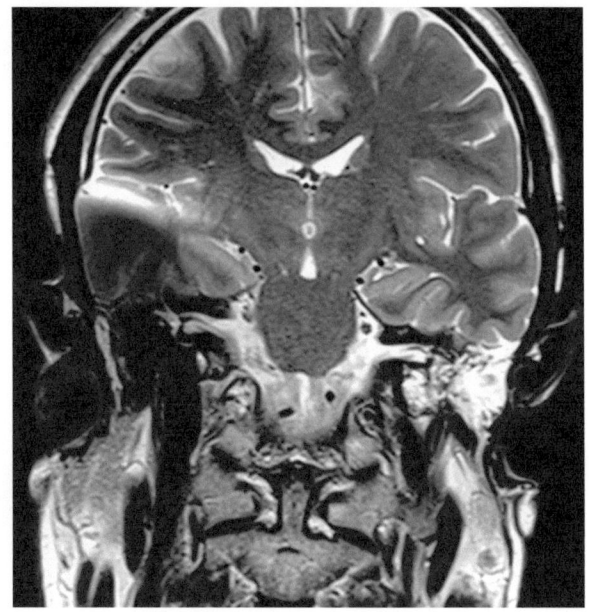

Fig. 14.7 Same case of Figs. 14.3, 14.4, 14.5, and 14.6. MRI T2 sequences with a CI in place after magnet removal. The temporal bone is completely visible with no distortion at all

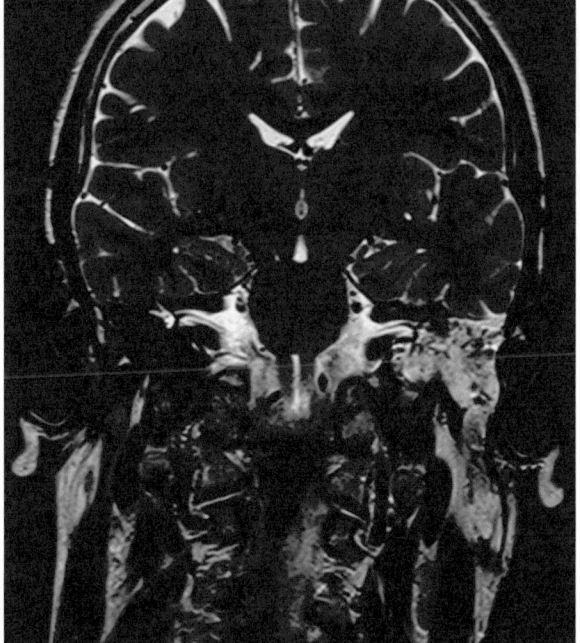

Fig. 14.8 CT scan 3D reconstruction showing bilateral magnet dislocation (white arrows) occurred after an MRI. The patient required a revision surgery bilaterally

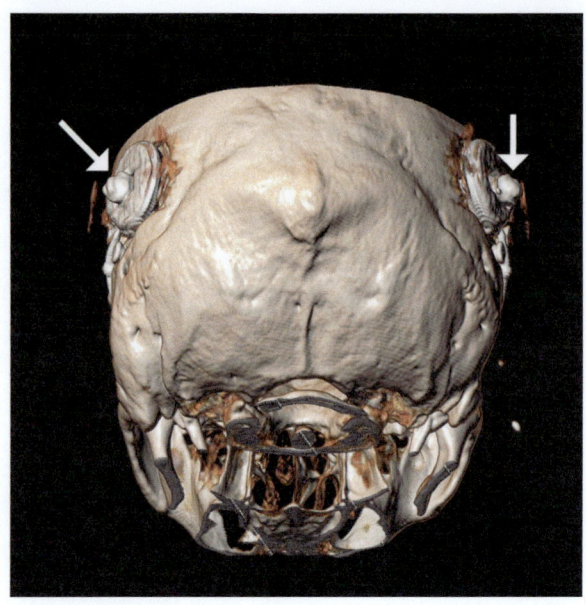

14.2 Complications

Patients treated for difficult cases may show the same complications occurring in the standard CI cases, plus additional ones related to the SP and/or the preoperative disease. In this chapter, there will be only an overview of these latter; their surgical treatment will be the topic of a further book.

Because of the deep retroauricolar retraction (Fig. 14.9) usually occurring in patients treated with the SP, a retroauricolar extrusion is much more common (Fig. 14.10), if the receiver-stimulator is not positioned far more postero-superiorly [5].

As in every case of SP, a breakdown of the blindsac closure may occur (Fig. 14.11), if the surgical technique is not perfectly performed, especially in the presence of infection [6].

A wrong execution of the blindsac closure if accompanied by an incorrect positioning of the connecting cable deep in the surgical cavity may result in an extrusion of the cable through the closure itself (Figs. 14.12 and 14.13). The medial cartilaginous layer of the blindsac closure is fundamental to reduce this problem [7].

A residual cholesteatoma may remain entrapped in a SP; because of the dead ear, it does not produce any symptom till reaching huge size, which means compressing the facial nerve or uncovering the dura, the sigmoid sinus or eroding the otic capsule (Figs. 14.14 and 14.15).

14.2 Complications

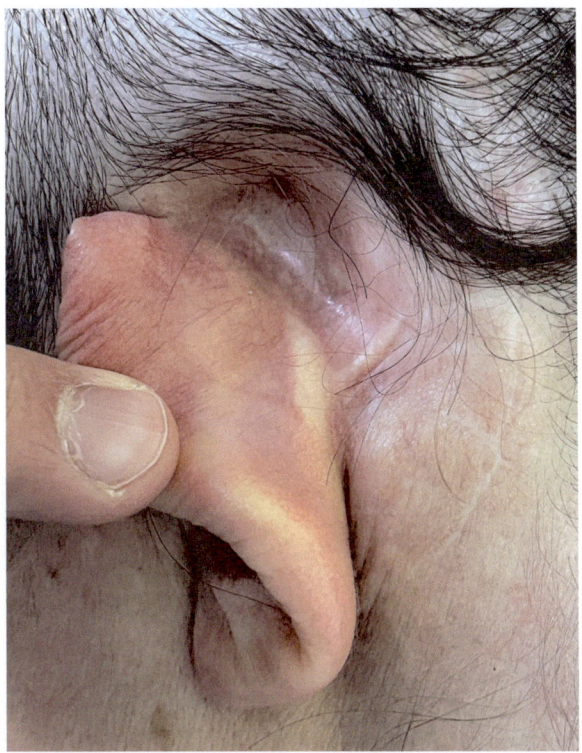

Fig. 14.9 A deep retroauricolar retraction is an usual finding after an SP

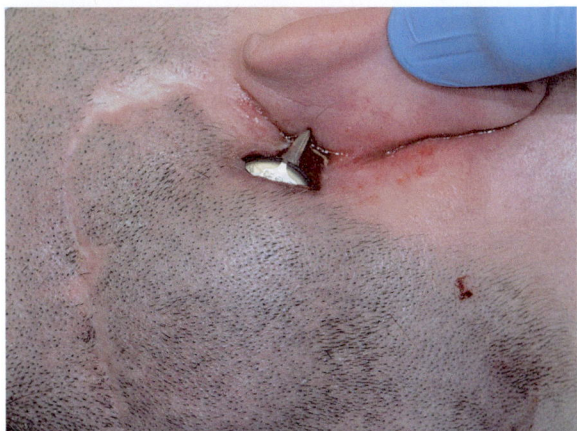

Fig. 14.10 Extrusion of the receiver-stimulator through the retroauricolar retraction is a common occurrence if not positioned far posteriorly

Fig. 14.11 Breakdown of the blindsac closure of the external auditory canal, completely replaced by inflammatory tissue

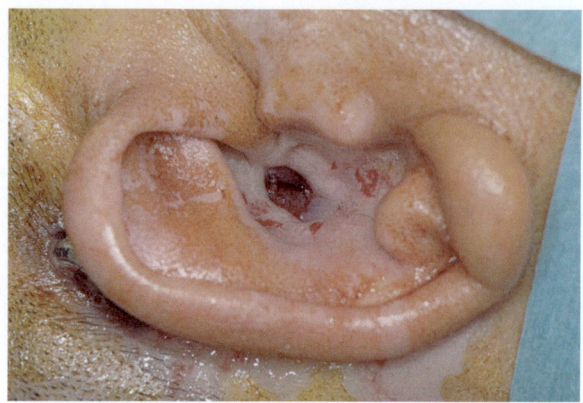

Fig. 14.12 Endoscopic image showing extrusion of the connecting cable through the blindsac closure of the EAC

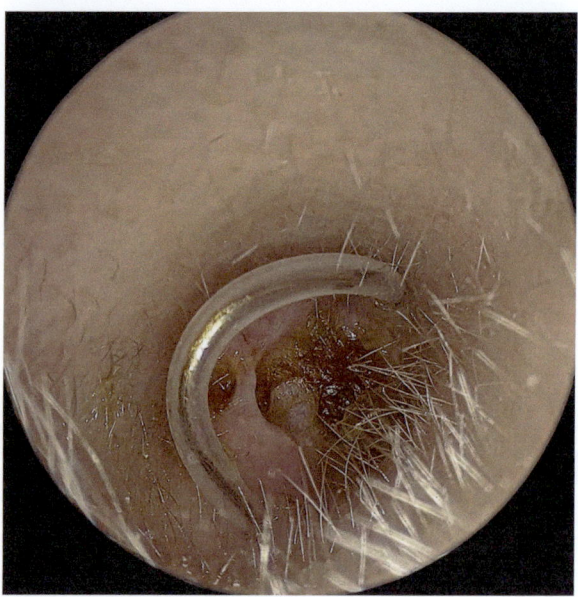

14.2 Complications

Fig. 14.13 CT scan of the same patient of Fig. 14.12 (extrusion through the blindsac closure)

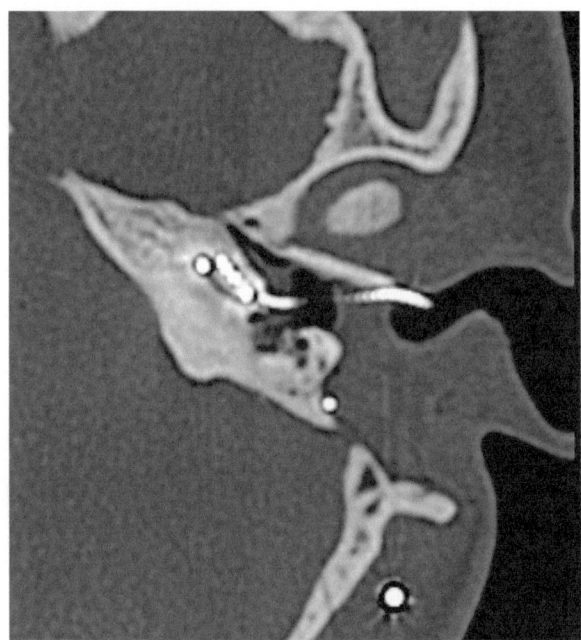

Fig. 14.14 CT, axial view, showing smooth erosions of the borders of the SP bony cavity. Note the lateral semicircular canal fistula (black arrow) as well as the exposure of the sigmoid sinus/posterior fossa dura (white arrow). The patient had been treated 20 years before and never underwent a radiological follow-up

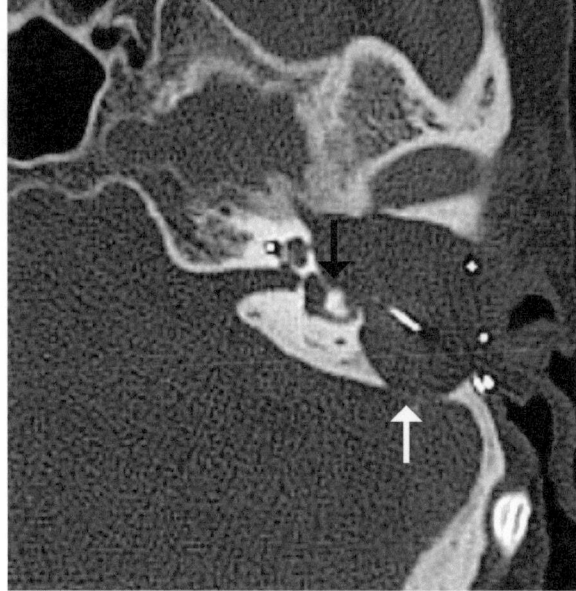

Fig. 14.15 Same patient of Fig. 14.14. The coronal scan confirms the presence of a huge fistula of the lateral semicircular canal (white arrow). In addition, a large tegmen erosion (black arrow) is also visualized. The axial and coronal findings strongly supported the presence of an entrapped cholesteatoma in the SP cavity

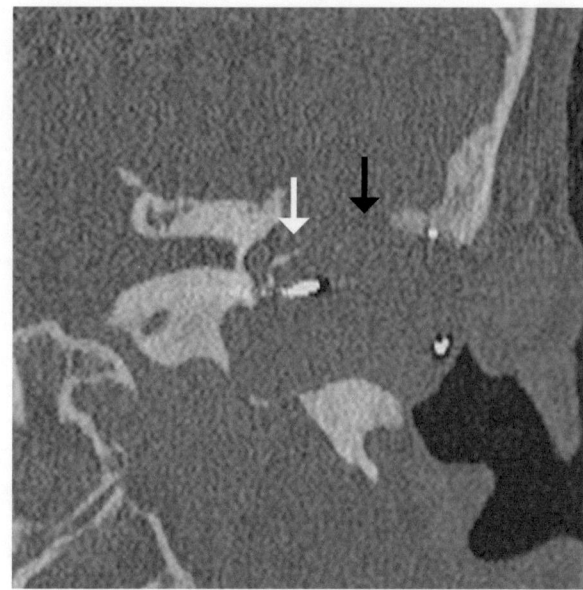

Fig. 14.16 Partial aeration (white asterisk) of the surgical cavity represents a relatively common occurrence after an SP. When it is confined to limited areas, it does not represent a clinical problem

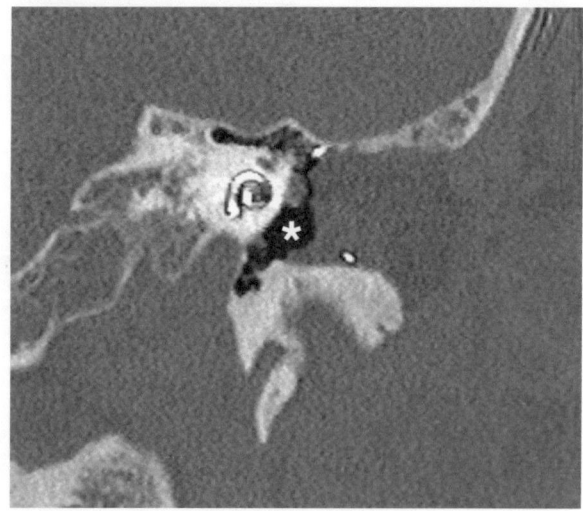

Another specific complication of the SP is represented by re-aeration of the cavity. In the majority of the cases, it is limited to the anterior mesotympanum and does not produce any symptoms/problems (Fig. 14.16). In rare cases, massive aeration can induce extroversion of the blindsac closure, if this latter has been medially not reinforced with a cartilaginous layer (Figs. 14.17 and 14.18). Even in this case, the problem is usually self-limiting because the entrapped air progressively reabsorbs spontaneously (Fig. 14.19). However, sudden opening of the Eustachian tube, often the result of strong sneezing, may produce clinical problems such as infection or partial array extrusion (Figs. 14.20, 14.21, 14.22, and 14.23).

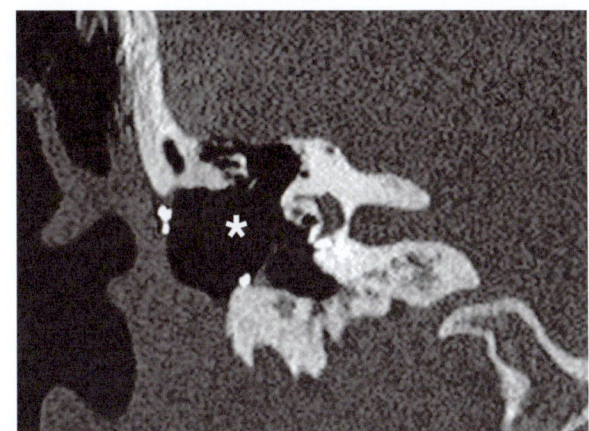

Fig. 14.17 Axial CT scan: a complete reaeration of the surgical cavity (white asterisk) has occurred; it was the result of a strong sneeze, with reopening of the Eustachian tube

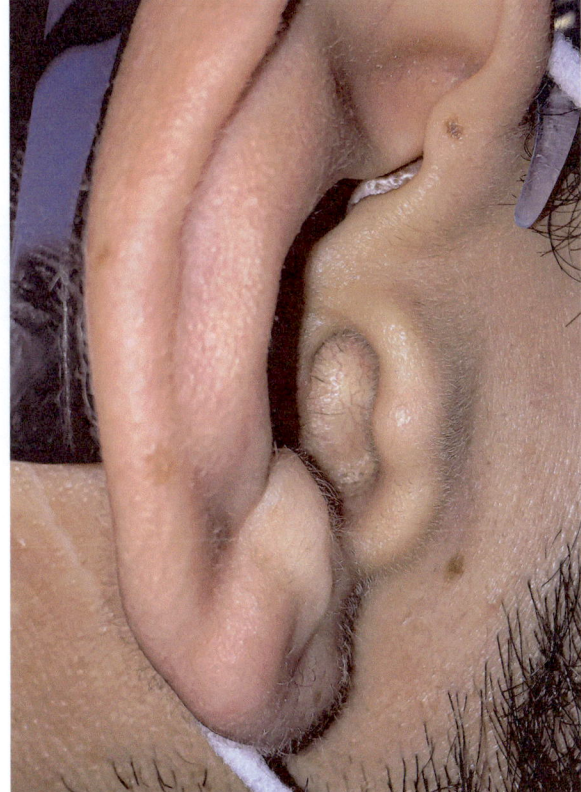

Fig. 14.18 Same patient of Fig. 14.16: the blindsac closure of the EAC (not reinforced with cartilage) has been extroverted by the air pressure

Fig. 14.19 Same case of Figs. 14.16 and 14.17. The air reabsorbed spontaneously in a few months. The blindsac closure returned to its original position

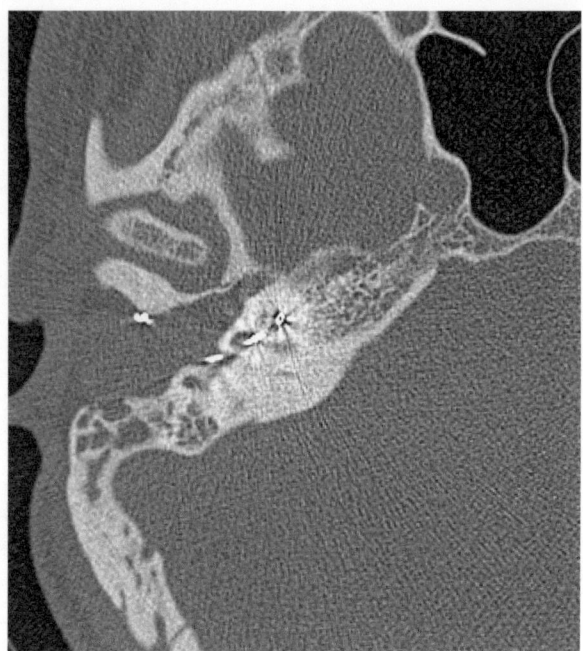

Fig. 14.20 Postoperative TC after an SP, showing a complete array insertion

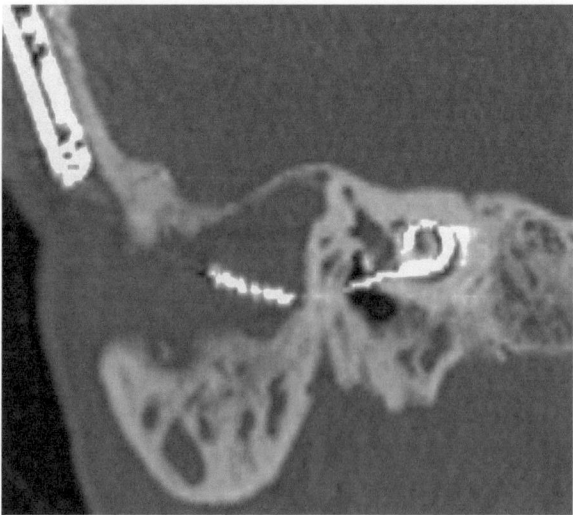

14.2 Complications

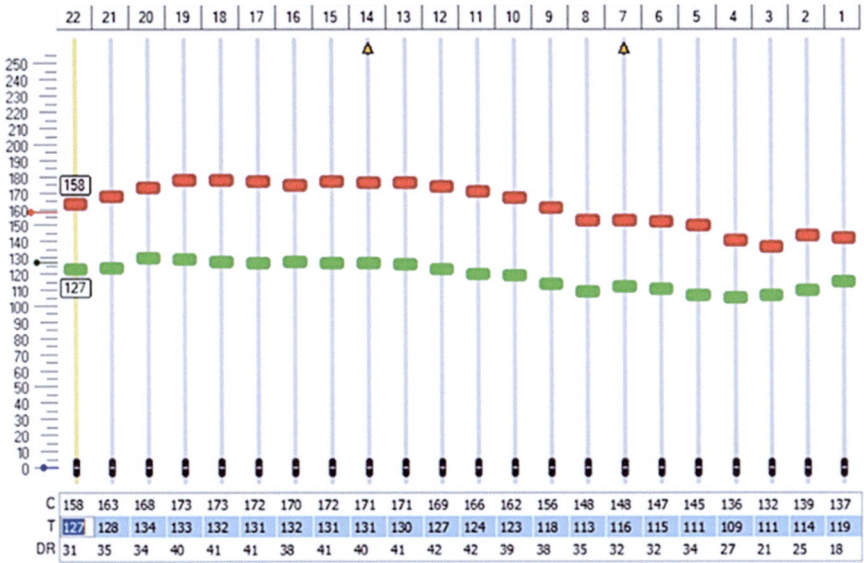

Fig. 14.21 The stimulation map of the same patient of Fig. 14.20 at activation confirms the complete array insertion

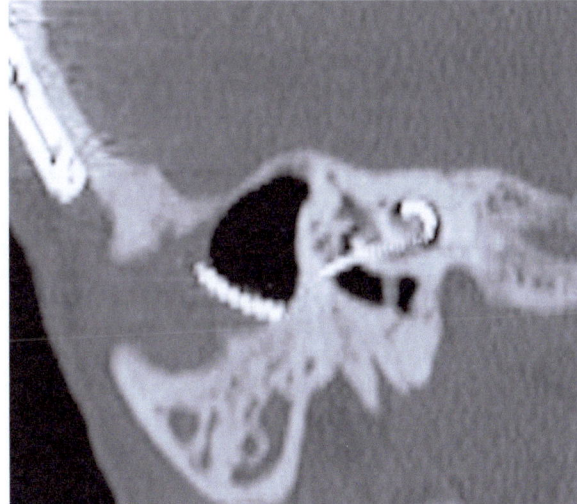

Fig. 14.22 Same case of Figs. 14.20 and 14.21. Sudden aeration of the surgical cavity has slightly pulled out the array (compare the position of the tip with that of Fig. 14.20). However, thanks to an "over-insertion" (performed by the authors whenever possible), the majority of the electrodes remained in the cochlear lumen

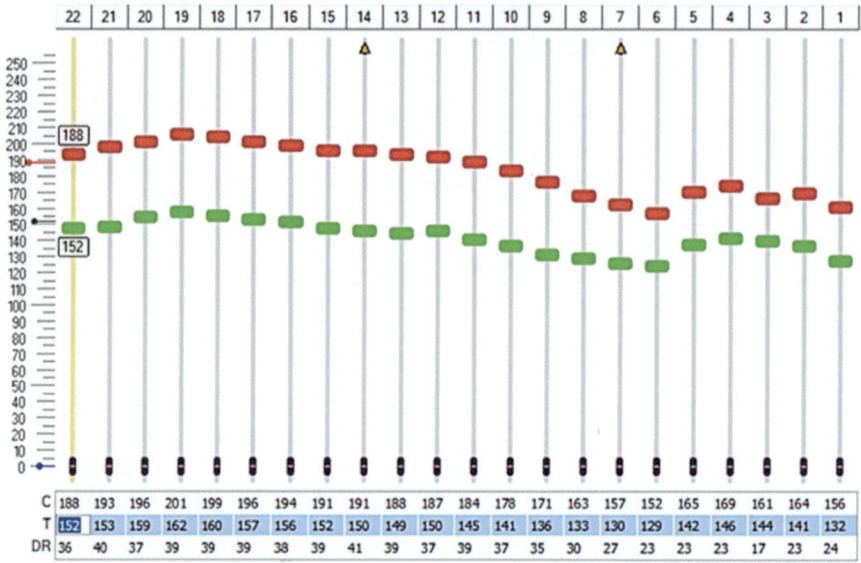

Fig. 14.23 The stimulation map corresponding to Fig. 14.22 confirms that all the electrodes are still active

References

1. Swartz JD, Loevner LA. Imaging of the temporal bone. New York: Thieme; 2009.
2. Sanna M. Surgery for cochlear and other auditory implants, 2015. Stuttgart: Thieme; 2015.
3. Pruitt P. Imaging of the temporal bone. DeckerMed Otolaryngol. 2020;
4. Vercruysse JP, De Foer B, Pouillon M, Somers T, Casselman J, Offeciers E. The value of diffusion-weighted MR imaging in the diagnosis of primary acquired and residual cholesteatoma: a surgical verified study of 100 patients. Eur Radiol. 2006;16(7):1461–7.
5. Coker NJ, Jenkins HA, Fisch U. Obliteration of the middle ear and mastoid cleft in subtotal petrosectomy: indications, technique, and results. Ann Otol Rhinol Laryngol. 1986;95
6. Issing PR, Schonermark MP, Winkelmann S, Kempf HG, Ernst A. Cochlear implantation in patients with chronic otitis: indications for subtotal petrosectomy and obliteration of the middle ear. Skull Base Surg. 1998;8:127–31.
7. Pepe G, Franzini S, Guida M, Falcioni M. Subtotal petrosectomy and cochlear implantation: revision surgery. Am J Otolaryngol. 2022;43(3):103333. https://doi.org/10.1016/j.amjoto.2021.103333.

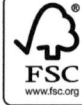

MIX
Papier aus verantwortungsvollen Quellen
Paper from responsible sources
FSC® C105338

If you have any concerns about our products,
you can contact us on
ProductSafety@springernature.com

In case Publisher is established outside the EU,
the EU authorized representative is:
**Springer Nature Customer Service Center GmbH
Europaplatz 3, 69115 Heidelberg, Germany**

Printed by Libri Plureos GmbH
in Hamburg, Germany